294
Current Topics in Microbiology and Immunology

F. Caligaris-Cappio and
R. Dalla-Favera (Eds.)

Chronic Lymphocytic Leukemia

With 35 Figures and 5 Tables

Springer

Federico Caligaris-Cappio

Department of Oncology
IRCCS San Raffaele
Università Vita-Salute San Raffaele
Via Olgettina 60
20132 Milan
Italy

e-mail: caligaris.federico@hsr.it

Riccardo Dalla-Favera, MD

Institute of Genetics
Columbia University
1150 St. Nicolas Avenue
New York, NY 10032
USA

e-mail: rd10@columbia.edu

Library of Congress Catalog Number 72-152360

ISSN 0070-217X
ISBN-10 3-540-25279-7 Springer Berlin Heidelberg New York
ISBN-13 978-3-540-25279-5 Springer Berlin Heidelberg New York

Editor: Simon Rallison, Heidelberg
Desk editor: Anne Clauss, Heidelberg
Production editor: Nadja Kroke, Leipzig
Cover design: design & production GmbH, Heidelberg
Typesetting: LE-TEX Jelonek, Schmidt & Vöckler GbR, Leipzig
Printed on acid-free paper SPIN 11017387 27/3150/YL – 5 4 3 2 1 0

Preface

Chronic lymphocytic leukaemia (CLL) is the most common leukaemia in the Western world. It is also the prototype of B cell chronic lymphoid malignancies. For a long time the Cinderella of lymphoid malignancies, CLL has now become the focus of major interest, and an increasing number of investigators from different areas including genetics, molecular biology and basic and applied immunology are becoming actively engaged in the investigation of CLL. Clinicians are considering CLL as a very interesting target of many projects that aim at translating the exciting developments of basic science into effective new approaches to the patient.

Many reasons account for this growing interest. First, both ethnic disparity and a strong familial tendency provide compelling evidence for a CLL genetic susceptibility. Second, the CLL cell has numerous features that cause uncertainties about its cellular origin. CLL lymphocytes are frequently self-reactive and produce polyreactive natural autoantibodies. They present many genomic abnormalities, especially in the advanced phases of the disease. Still, a molecular or cytogenetic abnormality unique to CLL has yet to be identified, and the CLL-gene(s) has become a sort of Holy Grail in haematological oncology. CLL differs from other B cell chronic lymphoid malignancies because reciprocal translocations that juxtapose immunoglobulin (Ig) loci to protooncogenes are exceedingly rare. Further, authentic CLL tumour cell lines have never been obtained unless infected in vitro or in vivo by Epstein-Barr virus (EBV). EBV-induced CLL cell lines are also extremely rare, as CLL B cells show a characteristic resistance to EBV-induced immortalization. Finally, only very recently, animal models that reproduce or mimic human CLL have been obtained.

Remarkable clinical properties likewise parallel these unusual biological features. CLL has a considerable clinical heterogeneity. Some patients present with an aggressive disease and a poor prognosis, others have an indolent course and a virtually normal life expectancy. Irrespective of these clinical differences, the cells from all patients have a common phenotype [$CD5^+$, $CD23^+$, surface (s)Ig^{low}], which is quite unique within the broad spectrum of chronic B cell malignancies. In addition, microarray analysis shows the cells to be surprisingly similar, confirming that CLL cells have the phenotypic profile of activated memory B cells. CLL patients present a severe immunodeficiency with hypogammaglobulinaemia, which progresses with advancing disease. The disease course may be characterized also by the occurrence of autoimmune manifestations caused by polyclonal auto-antibodies restricted to blood cell self-antigens that cause autoimmune cytopenias. These features suggest a complex disturbance of immunoregulation brought about by the malignancy.

All events that mark the natural history of CLL occur in tissues where the balance between proliferation and reduced apoptosis influences the clonal accumulation. CLL cell proliferation and extended survival are favoured by the leukaemic cell capacity to respond to the proliferative and anti-apoptotic microenvironmental signals provided by tissue bystander cells, such as T cells and stromal cells, through cellular contacts and soluble factors. Focal clusters of proliferating prolymphocytes and paraimmunoblasts (pseudofollicles) can be identified in the lymph nodes or the bone marrow. These focal B cell aggregates are infiltrated by T cells most belonging to the $CD4^+$ subset and represent the tissue proliferating reservoir of the downstream accumulation compartment that spills over and circulates in the peripheral blood.

The analysis of Ig variable heavy chain (IgV_H) somatic mutations which allow us to track the history of individual malignant clones to an in vivo activation triggered by the stimulation of the B cell receptor (BCR) discriminates two distinct CLL subsets, one with somatically mutated (M) and one with unmutated (U) IgV_H genes. The clinical importance of this biological observation is that the two subsets have a markedly different prognosis; U-CLL patients have a considerably shorter survival. This correlation links prognosis to biology and raises the question of whether and how the features of IgV_H genes and the properties of BCR may relate to the pathogenesis of the disease. The biased use of certain IgV_H genes, the existence of similarities among Ig rearrangements and the expression of gene products typically associated with B cell activation raise the possibility that an antigenic stimulation may be instrumental in the malignant cell growth. M-CLL are typically unresponsive to BCR stimulation in vitro similar to B cells that have undergone receptor desensitisation following chronic stimulation by antigen. On the other hand, though expressing germline IgV_H genes, U-CLL strongly respond in vitro to anti-IgM stimulation, suggesting that they carry a more competent BCR that remains able to receive signals for maintenance or proliferation.

All these studies have changed the perception of the disease called CLL and have transformed the little, resting, unremarkable CLL cell into an internationally acclaimed star that has become the subject of many reviews and journal articles. It is the aim of this volume of Current Topics in Microbiology and Immunology to convey the flavour of the exciting flurry of emerging results, going all the way from basic immunology into clinical application.

April 2005, Milan and New York F. Caligaris-Cappio, R. Dalla-Favera

List of Contents

List of Contributors

(Addresses stated at the beginning of respective chapters)

CTMI (2005) 294:1–17

B Cell Development and Its Deregulation to Transformed States at the Pre-B Cell Receptor-Expressing Pre-BII Cell Stage

F. Melchers (✉)

Department of Cell Biology, Biozentrum of the University of Basel, Klingelbergstrasse 50-70, 4056 Basel, Switzerland
fritz.melchers@unibas.ch

Abstract This chapter will review the scenario of normal B cell development—from the decision of a lymphoid progenitor to enter the B-lineage, over the stages of the generation of the repertoires of antigen-receptor (immunoglobulin)-expressing cells, to the response of mature B cells to develop memory and plasma cells—highlighting some of the cellular stages and the molecular mechanisms that can generate and select transformed states of cells. The scenarios for pre-B lymphoma (lymphocytic leukaemia) development are discussed in more detail.

1 Early Stages of B Cell Development

1.1 Ig Gene Rearrangements, Kinases and Cytokines

B cell development in mice and humans is ordered by stepwise, successive rearrangements of the immunoglobulin (Ig) heavy (H) and light (L) chain gene loci (for a more extensive review of B cell development, see Melchers and Kincade 2004). First, D_H-segments are rearranged to J_H segments on both alleles in both species. Very early stages of this cellular development are identified, first, by the onset of expression of the rearrangement-active genes RAG-1 and -2, and by the expression of the interleukin (IL)-7 receptor (in mice), and then by the expression of the genes encoding the surrogate L chain, V_{preB} and λ_5, by the IL-7 receptor and by the membrane-bound receptor tyrosine kinases, c-kit and flk-2/flt-3 (Fig. 1). Entry into these early stages of B cell development is controlled by the transcription factors E2A and EBF. During this very early development, progenitor (pro) B cells are in the process of D_H to J_H rearrangements, i.e. may carry one or even two H-chain alleles that are not yet D_HJ_H rearranged. We have called D_HJ_H/D_HJ_H-rearranged precursor B cells pre-BI-cells, and all earlier stages pro B cells.

Next, D_HJ_H/D_HJ_H-rearranged pre-BI cells enter V_H to D_HJ_H-rearrangements. These rearrangements are induced by removing the pre-BI cells from an environment of stromal cells in the B cell-generating organs, such as fetal liver during fetal development (of mouse and humans), and bone marrow (during fetal and adult development of humans, and adult development of mice). The specialized stromal cell environment is known to supply the ligands for flk-2/flt-3 and c-kit (in mice and humans), and for the IL-7 receptor (i.e. IL-7 only in mice; the cytokine for humans is, as yet, unidentified). Hence the ligands for the receptor kinases [stem cell factor (SCF) for ckit, flk-2/flt3 ligand for flk-2/flt-3] and IL-7 keep the cells at the pre-BI cell stage, inhibiting, in fact, further differentiation. It appears that the receptor tyrosine kinases control proliferation, while IL-7 inhibits differentiation. In mouse pre-B cell development, IL-3 can take the place of IL-7 at this stage of cellular differentiation (Rolink et al. 1995).

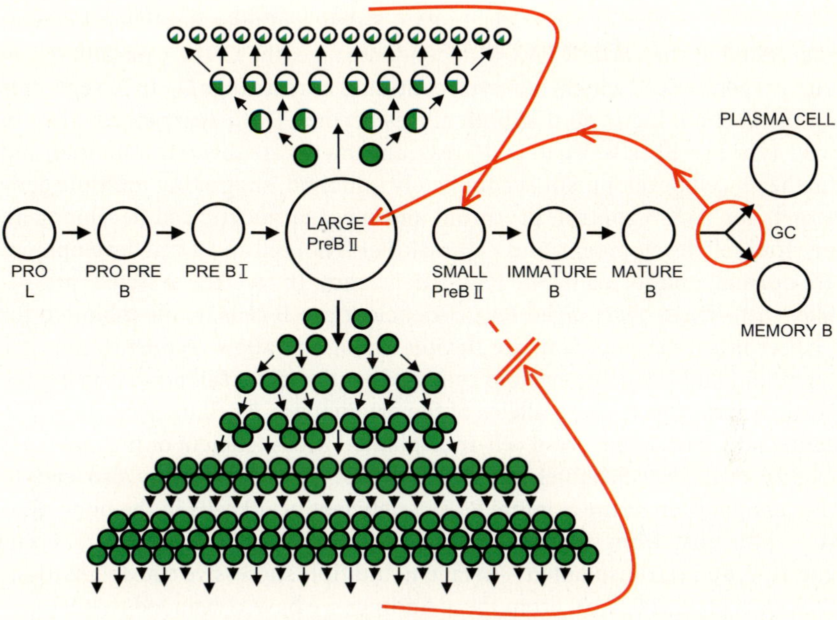

Fig. 1 Cellular stages of B cell development from early lymphoid progenitors to mature B cells, memory B cells and plasma cells. PAX-5-deficiency, induced either in the germline, or by hypermutation in antigen-activated, mature centroblasts and centrocytes in germinal centres (*GC*) inhibits the expression of SLP-65. SLP-65 deficiency, in turn, and involving IRF-4/IRF-8 and c-myc (see Fig. 2), blocks the downregulation of V_{preB1}, V_{preB2} and λ_5, i.e. of surrogate L chain. This deficiency prevents the normal cessation of precursor (pre) BII cell proliferation shown for four cell divisions (*top*) and maintains chronic, unlimited, preBcR-stimulated proliferation of pre-BII cells (*bottom*). In this proliferating state, further differentiation to small pre-BII cells is inhibited as long as preBcRs are expressed. PreBcR protein expression is indicated by the *intensity of green colour*. Note that while the proliferating pre-BII cells have the rearrangement machinery (RAG1, RAG2, TdT) downregulated, their neighbouring cell stages (pre-BI, small pre-BII) express it, conveying genetic instability

1.2 The Roles of PAX-5

The homeobox transcription factor PAX-5 begins its control of B cell development during the early stages of $CD19^-$ to $CD19^+$, partially to fully D_HJ_H-rearranged pro and pre-BI cells (Urbanek et al. 1994; Nutt et al. 1997, 1998). It continues these controls to late stages of B cell development and responses to memory B cells and plasma cells. In PAX-5-deficient mice B cell development is arrested at the earliest PAX-5-dependent stage, the $CD19^-$, flk-2/flt-3^+, c-kit^+ progenitor cell which, however, continues to rearrange D_H to J_H segments on the H chain locus, so that both alleles become D_HJ_H-rearranged—like in wild-type pre-BI cells. V_H to D_HJ_H rearrangements are severely impaired, and further B cell development is completely inhibited, suggesting multiple gene targets for PAX-5 control. Erythroid and megakaryocytic cell development, myeloid cell development, and natural killer (NK) cell and T cell development are normal, unaffected by the PAX-5 deficiency. In fact, the arrested, pre-BI-like, D_HJ_H/D_HJ_H-rearranged PAX-5-deficient pre-B cells, while inhibited for further B cell development, are flexible enough to allow reconstitution of T lymphoid and NK cells, myeloid cells and erythrocytes (all now carrying the D_HJ_H-rearranged H chain alleles of the original pre-B cell lines or clones) in sublethally irradiated, pre-B cell-transplanted RAG-deficient or normal hosts (Rolink et al. 1999; Schaniel and Melchers 2002). Transplantation also leads to the repopulation of the original PAX-5-deficient pre-B cells in the bone marrow of the host, from where they can be re-isolated, regrown on stromal cells and IL-7, and retransplanted—in fact, in multiple successive transplantations (Schaniel et al. 2002a,b). From these findings we have concluded that PAX-5-deficient pre-B cells have the properties of self-renewal, proper homing to the original sites in the body, pluripotency of haematopoietic differentiation and long-term reconstitution potential—all properties of long-term reconstituting, pluripotent haematopoietic stem cells. However, since they do not protect a lethally irradiated host from death, they lack the complete set of capacities of haematopoietic stem cells—probably because the rates of differentiation into the different lineages of blood cells are not normal. The capacity of D_HJ_H/D_HJ_H-rearranged PAX-5-deficient pre-B cells to retain their phenotype when transplanted into the bone marrow of a host, to display haematopoietic pluripotency and to show long-term reconstitution capacities have all been taken as evidence for plasticity, if not retrodifferentiation of these precursor cells.

1.3 The Pre-B Cell Receptor

Upon differentiation, i.e. entry into V_H to D_HJ_H rearrangements, the resulting pre-BII cells begin to proliferate whenever the $V_HD_HJ_H$ rearrangement has been productive (i.e. in-frame) and a μH chain has been made from this productively rearranged H chain allele, which can pair with surrogate L chain to form a pre-B cell receptor (preBcR) on the surface (for a review see Melchers

1999; Melchers et al. 2000). These pro BII cells, now large, because in cell cycle, will enter between 2 and 7 cell divisions, depending on the fitness of the μH chains to pair with the SL chain. The expression of the RAG genes is downregulated, so that further V_H to D_HJ_H rearrangements can no longer occur.

The preBcR performs at least two important functions in B cell development at the transition from pre-BI to large pre-BII cells. First, it signals—via $Ig_\alpha/Ig\beta$ and syk—proliferation of the large pre-BII cells. Second, it signals—again via Ig_α/Ig_β and syk, as well as via SLP-65 (BLNK, BASH)—the downregulation of expression of the genes encoding the surrogate L chain, i.e. of V_{preB} and λ_5. Hence, only the intracellular pool of surrogate L chain produced in pre-BI cells prior to μH chain—i.e. preBcR—expression is available for preBcR formation during proliferative expansion of the pre-BII cells. Surrogate L chain protein, thereby, becomes limiting as the cells divide, leading to an eventual cessation of preBcR formation—in cells producing a well-pairing μH chain at later divisions than in those producing μH chains that only loosely pair with surrogate L chain.

Several mutant mice document these roles of the preBcR, displaying either a complete block or a severely reduced capacity to proceed to large pre-BII cells and B cell developmental stages and beyond. Thus, defective H chain gene rearrangements (in RAG $^{-/-}$, SCiD $^{-/-}$ and J_H $^{-/-}$ mice) defective preBcR assembles (in μ membrane $^{-/-}$) and defective surrogate L chain gene production (in V_{pre1}/V_{pre2} double $^{-/-}$, λ_5 $^{-/-}$, and $V_{preB1}/V_{pre2}/\lambda_5$ triple defective mice) block (for all μH chain mutants) or reduce to 2% of normal (for all surrogate L chain mutants) the B cell development (Shimizu et al. 2002). Mutants of the signalling complex of preBcR (in $Ig_{\alpha/\beta}$ and syk) also impair the development at that stage. Deletion of the non-Ig portion of the λ_5 protein, or substitution of the seven arginines by serines in this non-Ig portion also abolishes the capacity of the preBcR to signal (Ohnishi and Melchers 2003). It is expected that a ligand interacting with the charged arginine residues of the non-Ig portion, autonomously produced by the pre-BII cells or supplied by the surrounding stromal cells—such as oppositely charged heparan sulphate molecules (but not autoantigens—selection binding to the V_H-domains of the μH chains) induces preBcR cross linking and subsequent signalling (Bradl et al. 2003).

None of the mutants of the preBcR and its signalling complex described above, with the noted exception of the SLP65/BLNK/BASH deficiency, is expected to lead to a transformed phenotype of B cell progenitors and precursors, as they abolish normal pre-BII cell proliferation and do not lead to an aberrant phenotype in apoptosis or migration of the blocked progenitors.

1.4
IL-7 and Its Receptor

The transcription factor PU.1 is involved in the induction of the expression of the IL-7 receptor, a crucial step in the early choices of haematopoietic progenitor cells to enter the lymphoid pathways (DeKoter et al. 2002). The IL-7 receptor remains expressed in the B lymphoid lineage of cells until the pre-BII stage, where the preBcR signals its downregulation (Hayashi et al. 2003; Flemming et al. 2003). In vitro, IL-7 keeps pre-BI cells from differentiating further to pre-BII, immature and mature cells and, furthermore, prevents apoptosis of the pre-BI cells in the absence of stromal cells, which are needed for the continuous proliferation of these pre-BI cells (Rolink et al. 1991).

Deregulated overexpression of IL-7 under the promoter of the E_α gene of MHC class II in transgenic mice does not change the sizes of the progenitor and pre-BI cell compartments in bone marrow, as long as these compartments can further differentiate to B cells (i.e. in wild-type or λ_5-deficient, but not in RAG-deficient mice; Ceredig et al. 1999). However, in the periphery (e.g. the spleen) significant numbers of progenitors, pre-BI cells, pre-BII and immature B cells are detectable, indicating that the bone marrow has limited sizes of the precursor compartments, and IL-7 provokes spillover of overproduced precursors into the periphery.

The primary targets for transgenic IL-7 action should be the B-progenitors and pre-BI cells, but not the preBcR-expressing pre-BII cells. Hence, if this deregulated stimulation by IL-7 should ever lead to transformed cells, it should be these progenitors and pre-BI cells that could generate malignant variants.

1.5
Resting Pre-BII and Immature B Cells

The exiting of large pre-BII cells from the cell cycle as a consequence of the cessation of preBcR signalling induces a resting G_0 state of now small pre-BII cells. The H chain alleles in D_HJ_H-rearranged conformations have been closed for further rearrangements (called "allelic exclusion" of H chain loci)—but apparently not through signalling via the classical preBcR (Shimizu et al. 2002)—and L chain loci are now opened for V_L to J_L rearrangements. They are initiated as the RAG genes are up-regulated and the RAG proteins expressed again. They remain expressed in small pre-BII cells as long as no L chain, no fitting L chain, or an L chain contributing to an autoantigen-reactive Ig has been made. The continuous opening of the L chain loci and the continuous expression of the RAG genes allow the small pre-BII cells to enter secondary and subsequent L chain gene rearrangements which appear to begin at one of the two L chain alleles and are followed, if allowed, on the second L chain allele and on the L chain alleles (Yamagami et al. 1999). Only immature B cells expressing IgM on their surface are allowed to exit the primary lymphoid organ (in adults the bone marrow) and to enter the peripheral lymphoid system, usually first into the spleen. Hence, normally no surface-bound (s)IgM-negative B cells are found in the periphery.

This selection of sIgM-expressing B cells appears to indicate that the insertion of IgM, via Ig_{α} and Ig_{β} and connected to intracellular signalling cascades, might ipso facto be a signal for selection and survival, or that all $sIgM^{+}$ B cells must interact with an antigen to be selected. The latter is likely for those B cells, belonging to the BI-lineage, which might well be selected by low avidity interactions with autoantigens and/or foreign antigens in symbiosis will the organism, such as the bacterial flora of the gut. While immature B cells will high avidities for autoantigens present in the bone marrow, and later in the spleen, appear to be induced to apoptosis, i.e. are negatively selected, it is unclear whether immature B cells expressing sIgM without measurable avidities to autoantigens are selected to become conventional B cells. Equally possible is a polyclonal selection mechanism in which BAFF, a ligand belonging to the family of tumour necrosis factor (TNF) ligands and recognizing the BAFF-receptor on conventional B cells, but apparently not on BI cells, induces differentiation to a mature, antigen-sensitive, resting G_0 conventional B cell population (for a review see Mackay et al. 2003; Harless et al. 2001; Rolink et al. 2002a, b). In these mature B cells, the RAG genes are no longer expressed.

1.6
Mature B Cells and Their Responses to Antigens

The invasion or infection by a foreign antigen triggers first the activation of $CD4^{+}$ helper T cells by antigen-presenting cells, such as dendritic cells, in the periphery. The activated T cells then migrate into the peripheral lymphoid organs, where the foreign antigen also activates resting, mature B cells. Germinal centres are formed in which mainly proliferating B cells of centroblast and centrocyte phenotypes are found. After the occupancy of sIgM on the B cells, triggering of CD40 (a member of the TNF-receptor family) on B cells with CD40 ligand provided by helper T cells induces the expression of AID (activation-induced deaminase; Muramatsu et al. 2000; Revy et al. 2000: Arakama; Hauschild and Buerstedde 2002). AID then acts on Ig loci in three major ways. It induces hypermutation, mainly of V_H and V_L regions of the rearranged Ig gene loci expressed in the proliferating germinal centre B cell centroblasts. Second, it induces class switch recombination via s-regions. Third, it induces the replacement of a V-region-encoding segment of a rearranged Ig locus by another V-gene segment. As a consequence of these reactions, hypermutated sIg-expressing B cells, expressing H chain classes other than IgM, are selected by antigen for higher avidities and they become memory B cells and high-affinity antibody-secreting cells. Both types of cells acquire longevity (will half-lives of 6 weeks to years) and exit the germinal centre, apparently to lodge back in the bone marrow.

2
Genetic Instabilities During B Cell Development

Mutations in proto-oncogenes and tumour-suppressor genes change—most often in several subsequent steps—normal B-lineage cells to transformed malignant states (for a review see Küppers and Dalla-Favera 2001). These mutations are more frequent when cells enter genetic instabilities. In the case of B-lineage cells a first and second wave of genetic instability is induced in cells in which the rearrangement machinery (RAG-1, RAG-2, TdT) is active, i.e. in pro and pre-BI cells, not in large pre-BII cells, and then again in small pre-BII and immature B cells. The rearrangement machinery can be expected to generate abnormal rearrangements, i.e. translocations of the regulatory elements of genes expressed in a given B-lineage cell (often the Ig loci) into proto-oncogenes (such as myc or bel-2, etc.), or translocations that destroy the function of a tumour-suppressor gene.

A second wave of genetic instability is induced when mature B cells are induced via CD40 by CD40 ligand (most often expressed on $CD4^{+}$ helper T cells) in antigen-specific responses to express AID. AID mediates class-switch recombination as well as hypermutations in actively transcribed genes in the activated B cells, i.e. in centroblasts and centrocytes of germinal centres. Again, as the rearrangement machinery, AID has the potential to generate aberrant translocations. Furthermore, it has been shown that AID hypermutates not only the V-regions of rearranged, expressed IgH and IgL loci, but also other genes expressed in CD40/CD40 ligand-activated B cells, e.g. bcl-6 or fas/CD95 (Pasqualucci et al. 1998; Shen et al. 1998; Müschen et al. 2000). The process and rate of hypermutation appear dependent on the rate of transcription of a gene expressed in germinal centre cells (Bachl et al. 2001).

To establish partially or fully transformed states of B-lineage, cell mutations in these cells are expected to be selected in vivo for their capacities to:

1. Proliferate more extensively and in deregulated fashions
2. Survive for longer periods of time, i.e. to be anti-apoptotic
3. Arrest a cell in a given state of differentiation, i.e. to inhibit the normal capacity of such a cell to enter further steps of differentiation

4. Migrate to abnormal sites in the body, where abnormal selections for proliferation, anti-apoptosis and arrest of differentiation may be favoured

3 Quantitation of Proliferation and Apoptosis During Normal B Cell Development

Proliferation, apoptosis and arrest of differentiation are reasonably well-defined parameters during normal B cell differentiation, from early progenitors to resting mature B cells (for reviews see Rolink et al. 2001; Melchers et al. 2000), as well as during antigen-driven immune responses of mature B cells to memory cells and plasma cells. In the bone marrow of a 6- to 8-week-old mouse, approximately 5×10^5–10^6 progenitor B cells are followed by approximately 2.5×10^6 pre-BI cells.

Therefore, these cell compartments are only partially in cell cycle; their apoptotic activity is low. A burst of proliferation with between 2 to 7 cell divisions occurs, when the expression of the preBcR as a consequence of a productive $V_H D_H J_H$ rearrangement expands the B-lineage cells within the pre-BII compartments to 2×10^7 large pre-BII cells. This is followed by 4×10^7 small pre-BII cells. While the proliferating, large cells show no measurable apoptotic activity, the small, resting cells become highly apoptotic, so that their half-life in vivo and in vitro is between 2 and 4 days. The 2×10^7 immature sIgM$^+$ B cells are also resting non-proliferating cells and show a similarly high apoptotic activity: their half-life is also between 2 and 4 days.

Only 20%, i.e. approximately 1–2×10^6 cells per day, appear in the first peripheral lymphoid organ, the spleen. These newly immigrated cells are still immature, highly apoptotic and short-lived. While we cannot determine yet with certainty what happens to the remaining 80% of the immature B cells that do not make it from the bone marrow too the spleen, it is likely that a large part of them is negatively selected by interactions with autoantigens present in either bone marrow or spleen, inducing accelerated apoptosis of such autoreactive cells.

Another part of these cells, possibly also autoreactive but with lower avidities to autoantigens, might be positively selected into the BI compartments that populate the epithelia of the skin and the gut. They constitute half of all mature sIg$^+$ B cells found in the periphery outside the primary lymphoid organs. These BI cells appear long-lived, possibly because their continued interactions with autoantigens keep them in an "excited", yet not actively proliferating, but anti-apoptotic state. Hence, they are easily transplantable into secondary hosts.

Almost all of the 1–2×10^6 immature B cells that enter the spleen each day also develop into mature resting B cells. As a consequence, interactions of the BcRs with foreign antigen no longer lead to apoptosis or to selection into the BI compartments but, most often, to proliferation and maturation into Ig-secreting plasma cells and memory cells. The amount of antigen usually appears to limit the proliferation to around 10 divisions. Helper T cell-dependent stimulation, furthermore, induces longevity of the emerging memory B cells and plasma cells, with half-lives of 6 weeks and much longer. Hence, T cell-dependent antigenic stimulation of B cells is a process that induces anti-apoptotic mechanisms that can be viewed as a potentially oncogenic event.

4
Normal Arrests of Differentiation During B Cell Development

Arrest of differentiation during normal B cell development can be seen at four different stages. In the first defined stage, D_HJ_H/D_HJ_H-rearranged pre-BI cells are kept from further differentiation in vitro (and, most likely also in vivo) by interaction with an environment of stromal cells in the primary lymphoid organs, which provide kit-ligand (SCF) and IL-7 to interact with c-kit and the IL-7 receptor on the pre-BI cells to keep these pre-BI cells at this stage of development. Removal of the pre-BI cells from this environment induces their spontaneous differentiation to pre-BII and immature B cells.

In the second arrested stage, B cells reach a resting, mature, longer-lived state—characteristic of most mature, peripheral, antigen-sensitive B cells. Removal of such resting mature B cells from their natural in vivo environment does not spontaneously induce their differentiation. The third stage is very similar to the original resting state of a mature B cell—only that the B cell has now been through a (usually helper T cell-dependent) antigen-induced response, and has reached the state of a long-lived memory B cell.

The fourth stage is the final state of B cell development, the long-lived, Ig-secreting plasma cell. While pre-BI cells undergo a limited, controlled number of divisions, the three other states of arrested B-lineage cells do not divide.

5
Mutations Contributing to Pre-B Cell Lymphoma Development by Interference with the Downregulationof Pre-B Cell Receptor Expression

Transformation of the four stages of arrested cells is favoured by the stimulation of long-term, chronic, deregulated proliferation, as it may be induced under chronic inflammatory conditions by the environment or by mutations in B-lineage cells.

In the case of large, preBcR-expressing pre-BII cells, normal proliferation is limited by the amount of surrogate L chain available for preBcR formation in these cells. Downregulation of surrogate L chain expression as a consequence of preBcR signalling limits this proliferative expansion to between two and seven divisions (Fig. 1). Consequently, mutations that affect this capacity of pre-BII cells to downregulate surrogate L chain expression affect the proliferative capacity of the cells.

5.1 SLP-65 (BLNK, BASH)

Deletion of the gene encoding the adaptor protein SLP-65 abolishes the capacity of large pre-BII cells to downregulate surrogate L chain expression (Figs. 1 and 2; Fleming et al. 2002; Jumaa et al. 2003). This leads to continued preBcR formation in dividing large pre-BII cells so that, in fact, SLP-65-defective mice have a hyperplastic large pre-BII cell compartment. This chronic pre-BII cell proliferation is a breeding ground for secondary mutation so that, in a period of weeks, pre-B cell lymphomas (lymphocytic leukaemias) develop in these mice.

5.2 Deregulated Expression of Surrogate L Chain

It is predictable from these findings, but has yet to be explored experimentally, that constitutive expression of the V_{preB} and λ_5 genes (as transgenes made active selectively in large pre-BII cells) will yield the same large pre-BII cell hyperplastic phenotype, and generate pre-B cell tumours. It could also be expected that mutations in other genes that are active in preBcR signal transduction for the downregulation of surrogate L chain expression, will have similar phenotypes and pre-BII cell-transforming activities. Double deficiency in the genes encoding the transcription factors IRF-4 and IRF-8 is one such combination of transforming mutations (Lu et al. 2003). SLP-65/Bfk-double-deficient mice have a drastically increased incidence of pre-B cell tumours, indicating that Bfk may also be involved in signalling of the downregulation of the preBcR (Kersseboom et al. 2003).

5.3 c-Myc

Expression of c-myc is downregulated for the first time during B cell development as large pre-BII cells become resting, small pre-BII and immature B cells,

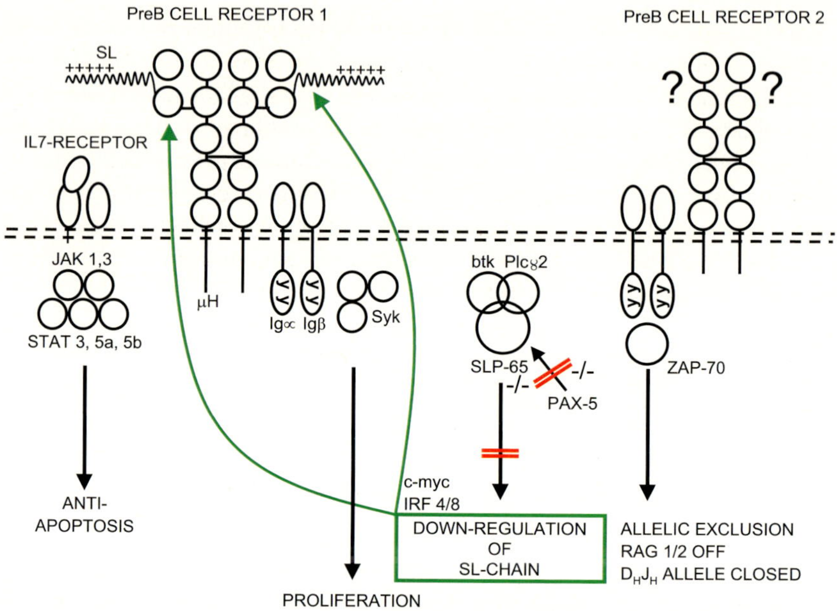

Fig. 2 Signal transduction in pre-BII cells. Four groups of functions of pre-BII cells are controlled by four, at least partially, different pathways. The IL-7 receptor (*IL7R*), composed of αand β chain and in association with Janus kinase (*JAK*)-1, JAK-3, signal transducer and activator of transcription (*STAT*)-3, STAT-5a and STAT-5b arrests pre-BI cells from further differentiation and prevents apoptosis in these cells. In pre-BII cells it looses these functions as its expression is downregulated. The preBcR, composed of H chains and surrogate L chain (*SL*) made of V_{preB} and λ_5 (containing non-Ig portions with positively charged (+) arginine residues in the λ_5-non-Ig portion is associated with Ig_α and $_\beta$. The ITAM-regions of Ig_α and $_\beta$, upon preBcR crosslinking, become phosphorytated, generating interactive sites with the tyrosine kinase syk. Direct, SLP-65-independent signalling via the Ras/Raf/MEK/ERK pathway induces proliferation, while association with Bfk in complex with PLC 2 and SLP-65 induces downregulation of the expression of V_{preB1}, V_{preB2} and λ_5, i.e. of surrogate L chain, and of the IL7 receptor. C-myc and IRF-4/IRF-8 are involved in this signalling pathway (see also the text). Finally, a H-chain-containing second form of a preBcR, devoid of SL chain, has been found in SL-chain-deficient preB II cells (Galler et al. 2004). It is likely to be involved in the signalling of allelic exclusion, i.e. of the downregulation of the rearrangement machinery (RAG1, RAG2, TdT) and of the closure of the D_HJ_H-rearranged H-chain allele preventing further V_H to D_HJ_H-rearrangements at that second allele. Mutations, which would abolish the signalling capacity of this second preBcR should lead to the premature reactivation of the rearrangement machinery, i.e. to genetic instability

i.e. as the proliferation-inducing signalling via the preBcR ceases (Winkler et al. 1994). Transgenic expression of c-myc under the control of the heavy chain enhancer Eμ surpasses this downregulation of the endogenous c-myc gene, keeps c-myc upregulated and, again, leads to large pre-BII cell hyperplasia and to the eventual development of B-lineage tumours. The phenotype of these tumours, at the time, could not be identified precisely, but it is likely that many of them are of lymphocytic leukaemia (pre-B cell-) type (Adams et al. 1985). These results suggest that c-myc is involved in signal transduction via the preBcR directly.

5.4 PAX-5

Finally the homeobox transcription factor PAX-5 has been shown to control B cell development at various subsequent stages of B cell development (Busslinger 2004). Its expression negatively influences myeloid cell development [by inhibiting e.g. the expression of the granulocyte-macrophage colony stimulating factor (GM-CSF) receptor] while it induces B cell development in sequence to EBF and E2A. PAX-5 deficiency arrests B cell development at the transition of ckit$^+$ flk-2/flt-3+ pro B cells to ckit$^+$ flk-2/flt-3$^-$ pre-BI cells, thereby either retaining or inducing these PAX-5-deficient pre-B cells to differentiate, under the appropriate environmental stimulations, to T and NK lymphoid, myeloid, erythroid and even haematopoietic stem cell development. The block of B cell development, induced by PAX-5-deficiency, must be the result of changes of expressions of a series of genes active in B cell development. Among them, and near the block of cellular development, is the inability to express the gene encoding the adaptor protein SLP-65, which signals the downregulation of surrogate L chain, hence of the preBcR (Schebesk et al. 2002). Consequently, PAX-5 deficiency might induce a large pre-BII hyperplastic state with the potential to develop pre-B cells lymphomas, unless other target genes for PAX-5 also regulate pre-B cell proliferation.

In this scenario of pre-B cell development, it is very intriguing that the deletion of PAX-5 by Cre in mature B cells of mice with a F-lox-ed PAX-5 locus induces retrodifferentiation of the mature, sIg$^+$ B cells to sIg$^+$/preBcR$^+$-double positive pre-B cells, probably because all the stages, from large to small pre-BII and from immature and to mature B cells, are controlled by PAX-5 (M. Busslinger, personal communication, 13th International Congress of Immunology, Montreal, Canada). When the Cre-treated, PAX-5- deleted B-lineage (pre-BII) cells are transplanted into recipient mice, they develop again into (now sIg$^+$) pre-B cell lymphomas.

6 Speculations on the Role of the Germinal Centre, Hypermutating Genes with Retro-Differentiation Potential in B-Lineage Cells

These findings open the horizon on new scenarios for the development of B-lineage tumours, particularly of the earlier developmental stages. It is conceivable that the induction of AID expression and, hence, of hypermutation in mature B cells responding to T cell-dependent (i.e. CD40–CD40 ligand-induced) antigenic stimulation, leads to hypermutation not only in Ig variable V_H and V_L gene regions, as well as in the bcl-6 gene, but also occasionally in other genes that are actively transcribed in germinal centre responses, i.e. in centroblasts and centrocytes. An analysis of hypermutating genes in normal centroblasts shows that only IgV_H and V_L, as well as bcl-6 genes are hypermutated, in contrast so the malignant counterparts of centroblasts, the diffuse large B cell lymphomas (Pasqualucci et al. 2001).

In these diffuse large cell lymphomas, additional genes such as c-myc, pim-1, and PAX-5 appear hypermutated. Interestingly, PAX-5 often carries missense mutations. One might speculate that a double missense mutation on both alleles of the PAX-5 gene could induce a deficiency similar to the one created by the experimental Cre-induced PAX-5 deletion of the F-loxed PAX-5 locus, reversing those germinal centre cells back to an sIg^+/$preBcR^+$–pre-BII cell, which continuously proliferates due to its inability to downregulate the regained surrogate L chain expression. That could lead, again, to sIg^+/$preBcR^+$ pre-B lymphomas, as one uncharacteristic subtype of diffuse large cell lymphomas.

In conclusion, our advanced knowledge of the cellular stages and the molecular mechanism of B cell development, notably also of early precursor B cell stages, have deepened our understanding of the possible scenarios of transformed and malignant cell development within the B cell lineage.

References

Adams JM, Harris AW, Pinkert CA, Corcoran LM, Alexander WS, Cory S, Palmiter RD, Brinster RL (1985) The c-myc oncogene driven by immunoglobulin enhancers induces lymphoid malignancy in transgenic mice. Nature 318:533–538

Arakawa H, Hauschild J, Buerstedde JM (2002) Requirement of the activation-induced deaminase (AID) gene for immunoglobulin gene conversion. Science 295:1301–1306

Bachl J, Carlson C, Gray-Schopfer V, Dessing M, Olsson C (2001) Increased transcription levels induce higher mutation rates in a hypermutating cell line. J Immunol 166:5051–5057

Bradl H, Wittmann J, Milius D, Vettermann C, Jack HM (2003) Interaction of murine precursor B cell receptor with stroma cells is controlled by the unique tail of lambda 5 and stroma cell-associated heparan sulfate. J Immunol 171:2338–2348

Busslinger M (2004) PAX-5 in B cell development. Annu Rev Immunol 22:55–79

Ceredig R, Andersson J, Melchers F, Rolink A (1999) Effect of deregulated IL-7 transgene expression on B lymphocyte development in mice expressing mutated pre-B cell receptors. Eur J Immunol 29:2797–2807

DeKoter RP, Lee HJ, Singh H (2002) PU.1 regulates expression of the interleukin-7 receptor in lymphoid progenitors. Immunity 16:297–309

Flemming A, Brummer T, Reth M, Jumaa H (2003) The adaptor protein SLP-65 acts as a tumor suppressor that limits pre-B cell expansion. Nat Immunol 4:38–43

Harless SM, Lentz VM, Sah AP, Hsu BL, Clise-Dwyer K, Hilbert DM, Hayes CE, Cancro MP (2001) Competition for BLyS-mediated signaling through Bcmd/BR3 regulates peripheral B lymphocyte numbers. Curr Biol 11:1986–1989

Hayashi K, Yamamoto M, Nojima T, Goitsuka R, Kitamura D (2003) Distinct signaling requirements for Dmu selection, IgH allelic exclusion, pre-B cell transition, and tumor suppression in B cell progenitors. Immunity 18:825–836

Jumaa H, Bossaller L, Portugal K, Storch B, Lotz M, Flemming A, Schrappe M, Postila V, Riikonen P, Pelkonen J, Niemeyer CM, Reth M (2003) Deficiency of the adaptor SLP-65 in pre-B-cell acute lymphoblastic leukaemia. Nature 423:452–456

Kersseboom R, Middendorp S, Dingjan GM, Dahlenborg K, Reth M, Jumaa H, Hendriks RW (2003) Bruton's tyrosine kinase cooperates with the B cell linker protein SLP-65 as a tumor suppressor in Pre-B cells. J Exp Med 198:91–98

Kuppers R, Dalla-Favera R (2001) Mechanisms of chromosomal translocations in B cell lymphomas. Oncogene 20:5580–5594 [review]

Lu R, Medina KL, Lancki DW, Singh H (2003) IRF-4,8 orchestrate the pre-B-to-B transition in lymphocyte development. Genes Dev 17:1703–1708

Mackay F, Schneider P, Rennert P, Browning J (2003) BAFF and APRIL: a tutorial on B cell survival. Annu Rev Immunol 21:231–264

Melchers F (1999) Fit for life in the immune system? Surrogate L chain tests H chains that test L chains. Proc Natl Acad Sci USA 96:2571–2573

Melchers F, Kincade P (2004) Early B cell development to a mature, antigen-sensitive cell. In: Alt FW, Honjo T, Neuberger M (eds) Molecular biology of B cells. Elsevier Science (USA), pp 101–126

Melchers F, Ten Boekel E, Seidl TH, Kong XC, Yamagami T, Ohnishi K, Shimizu T, Rolink AG, Andersson J (2000) Repertoire selection by pre-B-cell receptors and B-cell receptors, and genetic control of B-cell development from immature to mature B cells. Immunol Rev 175:33–46

Mueschen M, Re D, Jungnickel B, Diehl V, Rajewsky K, Küppers R (2000) Somatic mutation of the CD95 gene in human B cells as a side-effect of the germinal center reaction. J Exp Med 192:1833–1839

Muramatsu M, Kinoshita K, Fagarasan S, Yamada S, Shinkai Y, Honjo T (2000) Class switch recombination and hypermutation require activation-induced cytidine deaminase (AID), a potential RNA editing enzyme. Cell 102:553–563

Nutt SL, Heavey B, Rolink AG, Busslinger M (1998a) Commitment to the B-lymphoid lineage depends on the transcription factor PAX-5. Nature 401:556–562

Nutt SL, Morrison AM, Dorfler P, Rolink A, Busslinger M (1998b) Identification of BSAP (Pax-5) target genes in early B-cell development by loss- and gain-of-function experiments. EMBO J 17:2319–2333

Ohnishi K, Melchers F (2003) The nonimmunoglobulin portion of lambda5 mediates cell-autonomous pre-B cell receptor signaling. Nat Immunol 4:849–856

Pasqualucci L, Migliazza A, Fracchiolla N, William C, Neri A, Baldini L, Chaganti RS, Klein U, Kuppers R, Rajewsky K, Dalla-Favera R (1998) BCL-6 mutations in normal germinal center B cells: evidence of somatic hypermutation acting outside Ig loci. Proc Natl Acad Sci U S A 95:11816–11821

Pasqualucci L, Neumeister P, Goossens T, Nanjangud G, Chaganti RS, Kuppers R, Dalla-Favera R (2001) Hypermutation of multiple proto-oncogenes in B-cell diffuse large-cell lymphomas. Nature 412:341–346

Revy P, Muto T, Levy Y, Geissmann F, Plebani A, Sanal O, Catalan N, Forveille M, Dufourcq-Labelouse R, Gennery A, Tezcan I, Ersoy F, Kayserili H, Ugazio AG, Brousse N, Muramatsu M, Notarangelo LD, Kinoshita K, Honjo T, Fischer A, Durandy A (2000) Activation-induced cytidine deaminase (AID) deficiency causes the autosomal recessive form of the Hyper-IgM syndrome (HIGM2). Cell 102:565–575

Rolink A, Kudo A, Karasuyama H, Kikuchi Y, Melchers F (1991) Long-term proliferating early pre B cell lines and clones with the potential to develop to surface Ig-positive, mitogen reactive B cells in vitro and in vivo. EMBO J 10:327–336

Rolink A, Ghia P, Grawunder U, Haasner D, Karasuyama H, Kalberer C, Winkler T, Melchers F (1995) In-vitro analyses of mechanisms of B-cell development. Semin Immunol 7:155–167 [review]

Rolink AG, Nutt SL, Melchers F, Busslinger M (1999) Long-term in vivo reconstitution of T-cell development by Pax5-deficient B-cell progenitors. Nature 401:603–606

Rolink AG, Schaniel C, Andersson J, Melchers F (2001) Selection events operating at various stages in B cell development. Curr Opin Immunol 13:202–207 [review]

Rolink AG, Schaniel C, Melchers F (2002a) Stability and plasticity of wild-type and PAX-5-deficient precursor B cells. Immunol Rev 187:87–95 [review]

Rolink AG, Tschopp J, Schneider P, Melchers F (2002b) BAFF is a survival and maturation factor for mouse B cells. Eur J Immunol 32:2004–2010

Schaniel C, Bruno L, Melchers F, Rolink AG (2002a) Multiple hematopoietic cell lineages develop in vivo from transplanted Pax5-deficient pre-B I-cell clones. Blood 99:472–478

Schaniel C, Gottar M, Roosnek E, Melchers F, Rolink AG (2002b) Extensive in vivo self-renewal, long-term reconstitution capacity, and hematopoietic multipotency of Pax5-deficient precursor B-cell clones. Blood 99:2760–2766

Schebesta M, Pfeffer PL, Busslinger M (2002) Control of preBcR signalling by PAX-5-dependent activation of the BLNK gene. Immunity 17:473–485

Shen HM, Peters A, Baron B, Zhu X, Storb U (1998) Mutation of BCL-6 gene in normal B cells by the process of somatic hypermutation of Ig genes. Science 280:1750–1752

Shimizu T, Mundt C, Licence S, Melchers F, Martensson IL (2002) VpreB1/VpreB2/5 triple-deficient mice show impaired B cell development but functional allelic exclusion of the Ig H locus. J Immunol 168:6286–6293

Urbanek P, Wang ZQ, Fetka I, Wagner EF, Busslinger M (1994) Complete block of early B cell differentiation and altered patterning of the posterior midbrain in mice lacking Pax5/BSAP. Cell 79:901–912

Winkler TH, Melchers F, Rolink AG (1994) Interlenkin-3 and interlenkin-7 are alternative growth factors fort he same B cell precursors in the mouse. Blood 85:2045–2051
Yamagami T, ten Boekel E, Andersson J, Rolink A, Melchers F (1999) Frequencies of multiple IgL chain gene rearrangements in single normal or kappaL chain-deficient B lineage cells. Immunity 11:317–327

CTMI (2005) 294:19–29

Gene Expression Patterns in Human and Mouse B Cell Development

R. Hoffmann (✉)

Max-von-Pettenkofer-Institute, Ludwigs-Maximilians-Universität, Pettenkoferstr. 9a, 80336 München, Germany
r_hoffmann@m3401.mpk.med.uni-muenchen.de

Abstract B lymphocytes develop in the mammalian bone marrow through a series of developmental stages that can be ordered by recombination status of the immunoglobulin genes. Recent studies have combined RNA amplification by in vitro transcription with high-density oligonucleotide array technology to generate gene expression profiles of ex vivo isolated B cell precursor stages from humans and mice. Cellular differentiation through five subsequent stages of mouse B cell development involves differential expression of 10.7% of the 13,104 genes analysed, while between 2.8% and 6.8% change upon differentiation from one stage to the next. Early precursors express primarily genes involved in general metabolic processes, while B cell-specific functions are acquired in more mature stages. In human B cell development, pre-BI and small pre-BII cells express genes necessary for interactions with the respective microenvironments, while cycling, large pre-BII cells have a more cell-autonomous expression pattern. A direct comparison between human and mouse B cell development is hampered by the limited number of homologues that can be identified by reciprocal basic local alignment search tool (BLAST) searches of non-redundant expressed sequence tags (EST) clusters or of the available genome sequences. However, genes for which homologues could be identified that are differentially expressed during B cell development of both human and mouse have very similar expression patterns in the two species, are often expressed in large pre-BII cells, and are involved in DNA replication and cell-cycle regulation. Many more genes with homologous sequences, however, are differentially expressed during B cell development of only one species, indicating that genes can be used in different functional contexts even when the sequence is conserved. This implies that care should be taken with the interpretation of gene expression data from model organisms.

1
An Introduction to B Cell Development and Array Technology

B cells develop in the mammalian bone marrow through a series of progenitor and precursor stages that can be ordered by the rearrangement status of the immunoglobulin heavy and light chain genes. These cellular differentiation stages express stage- and lineage-specific surface markers. Five cell populations that follow each other in progressive differentiation in the mouse can be identified and sorted by fluorescence-activated cell sorting (FACS): (1) heavy (H) chain D_H-J_H rearranged, c-kit$^+$CD25$^-$ cycling pre-BI cells; (2) $V_HD_HJ_H$-rearranged, c-kit-CD25$^+$ cycling large pre-BII cells; (3) $V_HD_HJ_H$- and V_LJ_L-rearranged c-kit-CD25$^+$ resting small pre-BII cells; (4) surface (s)IgM$^+$ resting immature; and (5) sIgM$^+$IgD$^+$ resting mature B cells [20]. The earliest committed precursors, pre-BI cells, express the surrogate light chain encoded by *vpreb* and *λ5* genes [13] and the rearrangement machinery encoded by the *rag1*, *rag2* [8] and *tdt* [18] genes. As soon as one allele has been productively rearranged, somatic recombination is stopped, preventing additional rearrangements on the second allele. This process is termed allelic exclusion [18]. The μ heavy chain derived from a productively $V_HD_HJ_H$-rearranged IgH chain locus has to pair with the surrogate light chain to form a pre-B cell receptor (BCR) on the surface of large pre-BII cell [23]. Expression of the surrogate light chain and of the rearrangement machinery is then turned off [8]. The pre-BCR induces two to five divisions of large pre-BII cells [21]. As the pre-BCR is diluted by these divisions, the cells come to rest as small pre-BII cells, the expression of the rearrangement machinery is turned on again and V_L segments are rearranged to J_L segments on the κL and λL chain gene loci. As soon as an L chain has paired with the pre-existing μ heavy chain, IgM can be deposited on the surface to give the cell the status of an immature B cell. Autoantigens select the emerging repertoire of immature B cells negatively to delete high-affinity autoreactive cells, and may also select positively to differentiate low-affinity autoreactive cells into the B1 cell compartment [19]. Immature B cells keep the rearrangement machinery upregulated to allow for secondary rearrangements at the IgL chain gene loci with which they can change, hence edit the specificity of autoreactive cells [25].

B cell development in humans is strikingly similar to that in mice, and corresponding developmental stages can be identified by analysis of immunoglobulin gene recombination status and expression of surface markers [6,7]. Cells at the earliest stage of B cell development in human bone marrow, corresponding to the mouse pre-BI compartment, are CD10$^+$, CD19$^+$ and CD34$^+$. They express TdT and RAG-1/-2 intracellularly, and the surrogate light chain component of the B cell receptor on the surface. The immunoglobulin μ heavy chain locus is D_HJ_H rearranged. The second precursor cells in line in the human are equivalent to mouse pre-BCR$^+$ large pre-BII cells. In human, they are CD10$^+$, CD19$^+$, CD34$^-$, surrogate light chain positive, and do not express RAG-1/-2. The IgH chain loci are productively $V_HD_HJ_H$ rearranged. Subsequently, the cells lose the expression of the pre-B cell receptor and become CD19$^+$, CD34$^-$, surrogate light chain negative, large pre-BII cells. These cells can be flow cytometrically distinguished from their surrogate light chain-positive predecessors. After exit from the cell cycle, these cells (now termed small pre-BII cells) upregulate RAG-1/-2 and undergo immunoglobulin light chain rearrangements.

With the advent of microarray technology, it has become possible to generate gene expression profiles of cellular populations on an almost genome-wide scale. For the generation of "high-density oligonucleotide arrays", single-stranded oligonucleotides (25-mers) are synthesized directly on a solid surface, using photolithography to spatially address the area of synthesis (feature) on a glass slide or wafer [5, 16]. Synthesis features carrying a homogeneous population of oligonucleotides are currently 11 μm in size, allowing for more than 1,000,000 features on a 1.28×1.28-cm glass slide. For every oligonucleotide that perfectly matches the target sequence to be analysed, a second oligonucleotide exists with a 1 bp mismatch in a central position. This may serve as an internal control for hybridization specificity. Since current chip types use 11 or more oligonucleotide pairs to interrogate a single transcript, a single array of an up-to-date layout allows for analysis of transcript abundance of more than 47,000 genes. RNA from a single sample is labelled with biotin and hybridized to the array, and a complex three-step staining protocol is used to stain the hybridized RNA with R-phycoerythrin. Inferences about differences in transcript abundance are made from the comparison of two arrays.

The analysis of such microarray data is a complex procedure. First, different arrays have to be normalized against each other to correct for systematic differences in fluorescence intensity. Next, the fluorescence values have to be translated into numerical gene expression values; this step also includes some means of background correction. Some kind of statistical test has to be applied to give a list of genes that are differentially expressed between the cellular populations analysed, and this list finally has to be interpreted in the biological context of the experiment. For each of these steps, several different procedures have been suggested by different researchers. For example, there are vastly different methods to normalize arrays against each other [2, 15, 22] and a multitude of statistical tests is available (some of them correcting for multiple testing [24], others not); even for the translation of fluorescence values into numerical gene expression data, different methods (with or even without incorporation of the fluorescence intensity of the mismatch probes) have been proposed [12, 15]. In a comparative study of 12 different procedures, we have shown that it is possible to vary the number of genes that can be detected as differentially expressed with a confidence of 99% by a factor of almost three by using different analysis procedures [10]. The field is evolving rapidly, and there is currently no consensus about which algorithms perform best. Thus, the single "true" gene expression profile can currently not be identified.

For generation of the data described here, we have analysed gene expression profiles from highly purified cell populations isolated ex vivo. This has been possible after novel strategies for mRNA amplification by successive rounds of cDNA synthesis and in vitro transcription have been developed and adapted to microarray technology, concurrently by us and other laboratories [1, 4, 17]. These studies, as well as our own results [9, 11, 14], show that the amplification procedure preserves the cellular gene expression profiles and does not result in significantly biased measurements of gene expression levels. Previously known expression patterns of genes involved in B cell development could be confirmed with the array analyses, and for a subset of genes, the array-based gene expression patterns could be confirmed on the protein level.

2
Transcriptional Profiles in Mouse B Cell Differentiation

The relative abundance of 13,104 transcripts was first determined in the five consecutive stages of mouse B cell development described above [11]. We determined how many genes change in expression upon differentiation from one stage to the next, i.e. between developmentally adjacent cellular stages. Between pre-BI and large pre-BII, large pre-BII and small pre-BII, small pre-BII and immature B cells, and immature and mature B cells, a total of 488, 885, 462, and 362 genes have a t-test p value of 0.02 or less and change at least twofold. The entire pathway of B cell differentiation, as measured by nonparametric multivariate statistics (Kruskal-Wallis test) with 98% confidence and by a factor of at least two, employs differential expression of 1,406 genes (1,204 genes at 99% confidence). These large numbers of genes were unexpected, and subsequent analyses had to be performed to make a biological interpretation possible.

First, the set of 1,406 genes was subjected to a hierarchical cluster analysis, in that genes with similar expression patterns were grouped together (Fig. 1). This analysis reveals (1) that, except for large pre-BII cells, all cellular stages of B cell differentiation express a specific set of genes (those genes that are upregulated in large pre-BII cells are already expressed at lower levels in pre-

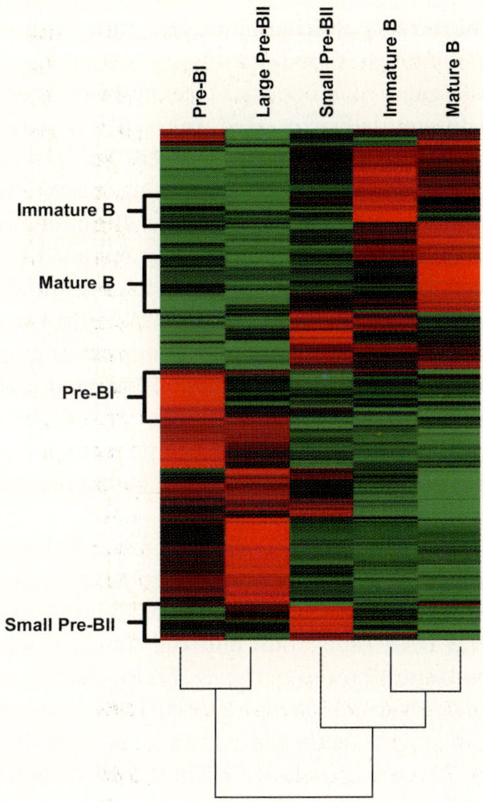

Fig. 1 Cluster diagram of 1,406 genes differentially expressed in five sequential stages of mouse B cell development. *Columns* correspond to cellular developmental stages (indicated on *top*); *rows* correspond to individual genes. Expression levels are colour-coded, with *red* indicating expression level above, *black* near to, and *green* below the row-wise mean. Clusters of genes upregulated in a stage-specific way are indicated on the *left side* of the plot. The *tree diagram* on the bottom compares gene expression profiles of the five differentiation stages, where *shorter branch lengths* indicate more similar cellular gene expression profiles

BI cells) (left panel in Fig. 1); and (2), that pre-BI and large pre-BII cells on the one hand, and immature and mature B cells on the other hand, have most similar gene expression profiles (bottom part of Fig. 1). By contrast, small pre-BII cells express one set of genes that is also expressed in earlier precursors, and a second set of genes that is also expressed in more mature precursors. This cell type can thus be considered "transitional" between these early and late B cell precursors. This is illustrated by the tree diagram on the bottom of Fig. 1, where shorter branch length indicates more similar gene expression profiles.

Second, the 656 genes [(as opposed to expressed sequence tags (ESTs)] among the 1,406 differentially expressed transcripts were functionally annotated by review of abstracts available in PubMed. This resulted in a definitive or putative annotation for 625 genes. Combining this functional annotation with the cluster analysis shows that a striking shift in functions of expressed genes takes place throughout B cell differentiation: pre-BI and large pre-BII cells mainly express genes involved in protein folding and degradation, DNA replication, cell-cycle regulation, and structural components of chromatin and of the cytoskeleton. By contrast, immature and mature B cells express genes involved in intercellular communication (secreted molecules as well as cell surface receptors), transcriptional regulation, and cell–cell contact (adhesion molecules). Thus, the functional compendium of genes shifts from general metabolic processes to cell-type-specific functions throughout B cell differentiation.

The functions annotated to differentially expressed genes also allowed for the identification of candidate genes potentially responsible for known functional properties of these cell stages. Hence, in pre-BI cells, besides genes controlling general DNA replication and cell division, we found cytokine receptors (thromboxane A2 receptor *tbxa2r*, *FcεRI*, endoglin *eng*, the common beta chain of IL-3/IL-5/GM-CSF receptors, *c-kit*), cell–cell contact or adhesion molecules (*gp70*, *a-catenin*, *lectin L14*), and signalling molecules (*p116RIP*, T cell-specific clone U2, *tiam11* and *socs2*). These genes might regulate homing of Pre-BI cells to their specific microenvironment, as well as the proliferative expansion in response to stroma cells and interleukin (IL)-7 or IL-3, a feature specific for mouse pre-BI cells.

In large pre-BII cells, two types of the pre-BCR control several functions, like proliferative burst and allelic exclusion, as discussed above. Besides the genes regulating DNA replication and cell division, which are found expressed in these proliferating large pre-BII cells, a total of 23 signalling molecules are candidates for molecular modes of control of proliferation, downregulation of surrogate light chain and RAG expression, and modulation of chromatin structures and accessibility for rearrangements. A number of these genes (*cdc25*, *ect2*, *stk1*, *sak-a*, *nek-2*, *ran*) are known to transmit cell-cycle progression. Calmodulin and calmodulin synthetase are involved in Ca-signalling. The signalling functions of others (*PP2Abalpha3*, *citron*, *fug1*, *pLK*, *ayk1*, *pMELK*, *mkp1*, *stam*) remain to be elucidated. Accessibility of H chain alleles may be controlled by those differentially expressed genes of large pre-BII cells that are involved in heterochromatin formation: *modifier-1*, the SWI/SNF complex, which modifies locus accessibility, and the histone acetylation-dependent transcriptional regulation by the retinoblastoma-binding proteins RbAp46 and RbAp48.

Small pre-BII cells exit the cell cycle and become small and resting. Two pathways leading to cell-cycle arrest can be deduced from our analyses. First, MyD118 (expressed in small pre-BII cells) and EAT/MCL-1 (expressed from immature B cells onwards) could inactivate proliferating-cell nuclear antigen (PCNA; a major cell-cycle regulator expressed in pre-BI and large pre-BII cells) by heterodimerization. Second, cdc25 is phosphorylated by the DNA-damage inducible kinase chk-1, which generates a 14-3-3 binding site. Binding of 14-3-3, expressed in small pre-BII cells, to cdc25, in turn, renders cdc25 inactive, blocking cell-cycle progression.

Immature B cells are characterized by a high propensity towards negative selection by induction of anergy or apoptosis due to the occurrence of autoreactive Ig molecules on the surface of these cells. Consistently, many genes expressed in these cells mediate negatively regulating signals: *cd72* (a negative regulator of B cell responsiveness), *c-fes* (negatively regulates macrophage activation), *pac1* (dephosphorylates MAP-kinases), *pirb1* (ITIM-containing inhibitory receptor), *FCγRIIB* (inhibitory coreceptor for the BCR), *calcineurin* (a Ca^{++}-dependent phosphatase), among others. Mature B cells, by contrast, are characterized by expression of many genes with activating functions, like *annexin V*, *mapkkk88, tank*, *jak-2*, and *adenylyl-cyclase type VII*. Resistance to apoptosis is reflected by upregulation of *bcl-2*. Expression of the chemokine receptors *ccr7* and *cxcr5*, and receptors for interferon γ and TAP underline the activation-prone status of mature B cells. This propensity for cellular activation is, however, counter-balanced by the expression of some receptors for inhibitory stimuli, like *il10*.

3
Gene Expression Patterns in Human B Cell Development

As mentioned above, human B cell development proceeds molecularly very similar to that in the mouse. Due to the higher surface expression of the pre-B cell receptor on human pre-BII cells, it has been possible to separate the large pre-BII cell compartment into a more immature, pre-BCR-positive, and in a more mature, pre-BCR-negative sub-compartment. In these four earliest stages of human B cell development (pre-BI, pre-BCR-positive large pre-BII, pre-BCR-negative large pre-BII, and small pre-BII cells), 1,065 genes have been detected as differentially expressed using Kruskal-Wallis test statistics at a 99% confidence level (unpublished results); this compares to 563 differentially expressed genes in the corresponding stages of mouse B cell development.

More mature stages of human B cell development, isolated from bone marrow, were not available for analysis.

Figure 2 displays a hierarchical cluster diagram of the 1,065 differentially expressed genes in human B cell development. It appears that fewer genes are upregulated at two or more stages of human B cell differentiation than in mouse—the different precursor stages seem to express rather non-overlapping sets of genes. Upon functional annotation of genes from these patterns of expression, it becomes evident that many of the genes expressed in pre-BI cells are signalling molecules, cytokines, cell surface receptors, and other genes involved in intercellular contacts or cell-to-cell communication. By contrast, genes with these functions are often downregulated in large pre-BII cells. These cells express mainly genes involved in cell-cycle regulation or DNA replication, and the functions of expressed genes do not change substantially upon differentiation from pre-BCR-positive to pre-BCR-negative pre-BII

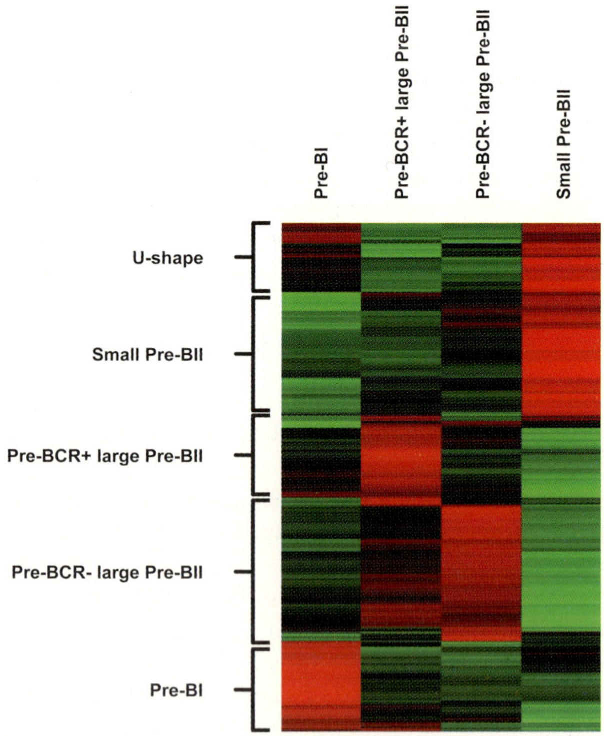

Fig. 2 Cluster diagram of 1,065 genes differentially expressed in four sequential stages of human B cell development. Graphical display as in Fig. 1

cells. Upon exit from the cell cycle and differentiation to small pre-BII cells, many genes are upregulated, these include again cell surface receptors, receptor ligands and receptor-associated signalling molecules. Surprisingly, small pre-BII cells re-express genes that have been expressed by pre-BI cells (U-shaped pattern in Fig. 2). This group of genes is particularly rich in signalling molecules and transcription factors. It is tempting to speculate whether these transcription factors regulate the same group of genes, or whether they are connected to different cellular functions, in these different cell types. Taken together, it appears that pre-BI and small pre-BII cells have the capacity to interact with their specific microenvironments. Large pre-BII cells have a more cell-autonomous gene expression pattern, and probably these cells are cycling independently from environmental signals. This is consistent with data from mouse B cell precursors, which indicate that the bone marrow microenvironment is not necessary for proliferation at this stage of development [21].

4 Expression Patterns of Sequence-Homologous Genes in Human and Mouse B Cell Precursors

A direct comparison of human and mouse gene expression patterns in hampered by the fact that homologous genes need first to be identified. This is most commonly done by finding sequence homologues between non-redundant clusters of EST or mRNA sequences from the two species by extensive basic local alignment search tool (BLAST) searches (NCBI LocusLink, TIGR EGO databases). More recently, the available genome sequences of mice and man can also be employed to identify sequence-homologous genes via reciprocal BLAST searches. With either one of these approaches, however, for only around 50% of all probe sets on the human and mouse arrays can a sequence homologue, which is represented on the arrays of the other species, be identified. This low proportion is in contrast to recent estimates from a comparative analysis of the human and mouse genome sequences, which predicted that 99% of all mouse genes should have a human homologue [3].

Among the genes that are differentially expressed in human B cell development, only around 15% have a sequence homologue in mouse that is also differentially expressed in mouse B cell development. The expression patterns of these genes are nearly identical between mouse and man. Many of them are expressed in large pre-BII cells and involved in cell-cycle regulation and DNA replication. This indicates that these genes constitute a core set that is essential for cellular replication, and thus well conserved both in sequence and in expression pattern among species. In contrast, a large proportion of differentially expressed genes in human B cell development, around 40%, have a sequence homologue in mouse that is not differentially expressed in mouse B cell development. These genes stem from a variety of functional classes. This shows that genes can be utilized in different functional contexts in different species, even when the sequence appears well conserved. Thus, we conclude that care should be taken when experimental results based on gene expression are to be transferred from one species to another.

References

1. Baugh LR, Hill AA, Brown EL, Hunter CP (2001) Quantitative analysis of mRNA amplification by in vitro transcription. Nucleic Acids Res 29:E29
2. Bolstad BM, Irizarry RA, Astrand M, Speed TP (2003) A comparison of normalization methods for high density oligonucleotide array data based on variance and bias. Bioinformatics 19:185–193
3. Waterston RH, Lindblad-Toh K, Birney E, Rogers J, Abril JF, Agarwal P, Agarwala R, Ainscough R, Alexandersson M, An P, Antonarakis SE, Attwood J, Baertsch R, et al (2002) Initial sequencing and comparative analysis of the mouse genome. Nature 420:520–562
4. Eberwine J, Yeh H, Miyashiro K, Cao Y, Nair S, Finnell R, Zettel M, Coleman P (1992) Analysis of gene expression in single live neurons. Proc Natl Acad Sci U S A 89:3010–3014
5. Fodor SP, Read JL, Pirrung MC, Stryer L, Lu AT, Solas D (1991) Light-directed, spatially addressable parallel chemical synthesis. Science 251:767–773
6. Ghia P, ten Boekel E, Rolink AG, Melchers F (1998) B-cell development: a comparison between mouse and man. Immunol Today 19:480–485
7. Ghia P, ten Boekel E, Sanz E, de la Hera A, Rolink A, Melchers F (1996) Ordering of human bone marrow B lymphocyte precursors by single-cell polymerase chain reaction analyses of the rearrangement status of the immunoglobulin H and L chain gene loci. J Exp Med 184:2217–2229
8. Grawunder U, Leu TM, Schatz DG, Werner A, Rolink AG, Melchers F, Winkler TH (1995) Down-regulation of RAG1 and RAG2 gene expression in preB cells after functional immunoglobulin heavy chain rearrangement. Immunity 3:601–608
10. Hoffmann R, Seidl T, Dugas M (2002a) Profound effect of normalization on detection of differentially expressed genes in oligonucleotide microarray data analysis. Genome Biol 3:research0033.1–0033.11
11. Hoffmann R, Seidl T, Neeb M, Rolink A, Melchers F (2002b) Changes in gene expression profiles in developing B cells of murine bone marrow. Genome Res 12:98–111
9. Hoffmann R, Bruno L, Seidl T, Rolink A, Melchers F (2003) Rules for gene usage inferred from a comparison of large-scale gene expression profiles of T and B lymphocyte development. J Immunol 170:1339–1353
12. Irizarry RA, Bolstad BM, Collin F, Cope LM, Hobbs B, Speed TP (2003) Summaries of Affymetrix GeneChip probe level data. Nucleic Acids Res 31:e15

13. Karasuyama H, Rolink A, Shinkai Y, Young F, Alt FW, Melchers F (1994) The expression of Vpre-B/lambda 5 surrogate light chain in early bone marrow precursor B cells of normal and B cell-deficient mutant mice. Cell 77:133–143
14. Kretschmer K, Jungebloud A, Stopkowicz J, Stoermann B, Hoffmann R, Weiss S (2003) Antibody repertoire and gene expression profile: implications for different developmental and functional traits of splenic and peritoneal B-1 lymphocytes. J Immunol 171:1192–1201
15. Li C, WH Wong (2001) Model-based analysis of oligonucleotide arrays: expression index computation and outlier detection. Proc Natl Acad Sci U S A 98:31–36
16. Lockhart DJ, Dong H, Byrne MC, Follettie MT, Gallo MV, Chee MS, Mittmann M, Wang C, Kobayashi M, Horton H, Brown EL (1996) Expression monitoring by hybridization to high-density oligonucleotide arrays. Nat Biotechnol 14:1675–1680
17. Luo L, Salunga RC, Guo H, Bittner A, Joy KC, Galindo JE, Xiao H, Rogers KE, Wan JS, Jackson MR, Erlander MG (1999) Gene expression profiles of laser-captured adjacent neuronal subtypes [published erratum appears in Nat Med 1999 Mar;5(3):355]. Nat Med 5:117–122
18. Melchers F, Rolink A (1999) B-Lymphocyte development and biology. In: Paul WE (ed) Fundamental immunology. Lippincott-Raven: Philadelphia, New York, p 183–224
19. Nemazee D, Kouskoff V, Hertz M, Lang J, Melamed D, Pape K, Retter M (2000) B-cell-receptor-dependent positive and negative selection in immature B cells. Curr Top Microbiol Immunol 245:57–71
20. Rolink A, Grawunder U, Winkler TH, Karasuyama H, Melchers F (1994) IL-2 receptor alpha chain (CD25, TAC) expression defines a crucial stage in pre-B cell development. Int Immunol 6:1257–1264
21. Rolink AG, Winkler T, Melchers F, Andersson J (2000) Precursor B cell receptor-dependent B cell proliferation and differentiation does not require the bone marrow or fetal liver environment [see comments]. J Exp Med 191:23–32
22. Stuart RO, KT Bush, SK Nigam (2001) Changes in global gene expression patterns during development and maturation of the rat kidney. Proc Natl Acad Sci U S A 98:5649–5654
23. ten Boekel E, Melchers F, Rolink AG (1997) Changes in the V(H) gene repertoire of developing precursor B lymphocytes in mouse bone marrow mediated by the pre-B cell receptor. Immunity 7:357–368
24. Tusher VG, Tibshirani R, Chu G (2001) Significance analysis of microarrays applied to the ionizing radiation response. Proc Natl Acad Sci U S A 98:5116–5121
25. Yu W, Nagaoka H, Jankovic M, Misulovin Z, Suh H, Rolink A, Melchers F, Meffre E, Nussenzweig MC (1999) Continued RAG expression in late stages of B cell development and no apparent re-induction after immunization. Nature 400:682–687

CTMI (2005) 294:31–49

New Insights into the Phenotype and Cell Derivation of B Cell Chronic Lymphocytic Leukemia

U. Klein · R. Dalla-Favera (✉)

Institute for Cancer Genetics, Columbia University, 1150 St. Nicholas Ave., New York, NY 10032, USA
rd10@columbia.edu

Abstract For many decades, B cell chronic lymphocytic leukemia (B-CLL) stood out as a B cell-derived malignancy that was difficult to position within the framework of the available B cell differentiation scheme: First, the histology as well as the immunophenotype did not quite resemble that of any normal lymphocyte; second, in contrast to almost all other B cell tumor subtypes, the immunoglobulin variable region (IgV) genes of B-CLL cases could be either unmutated or somatically mutated; third, the genomic lesions observed in B-CLL were markedly distinct from those of the other major B cell malignancies, which typically exhibit balanced chromosome translocations. Recent advances in the characterization of both B-CLL and normal B cell subpopulations by phenotypic analysis, global gene expression profiling, as well as extensive IgV gene repertoire analyses have shed new light on the phenotype and the cell derivation of B-CLL and provided novel hypotheses concerning its pathogenesis. Here we summarize recent work relevant to these issues and conclude that B-CLL may be derived from a cell that can be referred to as a marginal zone B cell. Moreover, we propose that the lack of chromosomal translocations in B-CLL may be related to their derivation from marginal zone B cells, since somatic hypermutation and Ig class switch, the processes that generate chromosome translocations in most germinal center (GC)-derived malignancies, are no longer active in marginal zone B cells. Also, we discuss similarities and differences between B-CLL and hairy cell leukemia (HCL) and suggest that also HCL may be derived from a post-GC memory or marginal zone B cell.

Abbreviations

B-CLL	B cell chronic lymphocytic leukemia
Ig	Immunoglobulin
IgV	Immunoglobulin variable
GC	Germinal center
MZB	Marginal zone B cell
MM	Multiple myeloma
HCL	Hairy cell leukemia

1 Introduction

B-CLL is characterized by the monoclonal expansion of mature, resting B lymphocytes that are present in the peripheral blood, bone marrow, and lymphoid organs, and by an indolent disease course that ultimately becomes lethal (Caligaris-Cappio and Hamblin 1999). In contrast to most other B cell malignancies, which typically show reciprocal balanced chromosome translocations, no specific genetic alteration has yet been associated with this disease (Döhner et al. 1999). The low proliferative rate of B-CLL cells and their prolonged life span suggests that a critical alteration might be a defect in apoptosis (Caligaris-Cappio and Hamblin 1999).

B-CLL has been the focus of intense investigations over many decades, and many studies revealed a number of surprising and unexpected findings in the light of previously obtained knowledge on healthy and transformed B lymphocytes. First, although based on the expression of the CD5 antigen on the tumor cells B-CLL had initially been thought to be derived from—namely the small subset of CD5-positive B lymphocytes (Dighiero et al. 1996)—the immunophenotype of the B-CLL tumor cells ($CD5^+$, $CD23^+$, $CD27^+$, and low levels of surface Ig expression) is clearly distinct from that of any known normal B cell (Kipps 1998; Caligaris-Cappio and Hamblin 1999). Second, the finding that B-CLL cases can express either somatically mutated or unmutated IgV genes (Schroeder and Dighiero 1994; Oscier et al. 1997; Fais et al. 1998)—and that those subgroups have a different prognosis, since the IgV gene-unmutated B-CLL cases show a more aggressive clinical course (Damle et al. 1999; Hamblin et al. 1999)—was surprising since the tumor cells exhibit a largely homogeneous phenotype. A proposed correlation between the expression of the CD38 cell surface marker on B-CLL cells and clinical course has been controversial (Damle et al. 1999; Hamblin et al. 2000; Jelinek et al. 2001; Hamblin et al. 2002), in part due to the fact that CD38 expression levels are heterogeneous within the same tumor case and may also change over the disease course (Hamblin et al. 2002). Third, IgV gene repertoire analyses early on suggested that B-CLL express a restricted set of IgV gene segments (Chiorazzi and Ferrarini 2003), a circumstance that invokes a possible role for antigen in the pathogenesis of B-CLL. This hypothesis found support in the high replacement to silent nucleotide exchange (R/S) ratios in IgV genes of somatically mutated B-CLL cases, which are indicative of antigenic selection (Fais et al. 1998). Finally, B-CLL exhibit various genetic lesions, mostly chromosomal deletions, many of which are specific and recurrent (Döhner et al. 1999). Most of those genomic alterations are not unique to B-CLL as they are frequently observed in other non-hematological tumors. There does not appear to be a strong correlation between a particular genetic lesion in B-CLL and either the level of IgV gene hypermutation or clinical course. Therefore, the level of IgV gene hypermutation appears as the best prognostic marker in B-CLL.

Taken together, the above observations pointed towards the existence of subgroups within B-CLL that may correspond to different B cell developmental stages. In fact, the B-CLL cases with somatically mutated IgV genes may originate from B cells that have undergone the GC-response of T cell-dependent immune responses in which B cells hypermutate their rearranged IgV genes to generate high-affinity antibody mutants (MacLennan 1994; Rajewsky 1996); whereas B-CLLs with unmutated IgV genes would be derived from the malignant transformation of antigen-inexperienced, naïve B cells. Although this widely suggested hypothesis (Oscier et al. 1997; Fais et al. 1998; Hamblin et al. 1999; Küppers et al. 1999) failed to explain the different clinical courses of IgV-unmutated and -mutated B-CLLs, it provided a reasonable explanation consistent with current concepts of B cell development (MacLennan 1994; Rajewsky 1996).

However, this hypothesis was challenged by recent studies on gene expression profiles and large-scale IgV gene repertoire analyses of clinically characterized B-CLL cases, as well as by new observations that emerged from studies on normal B cell subpopulations.

2
B-CLL Shows a Homogeneous Gene Expression Profile

Gene expression profiling using various gene chip “platforms” were performed by several laboratories during the last several years (Klein et al. 2001; Rosenwald et al. 2001; Stratowa et al. 2001; Dürig et al. 2003; Jelinek et al. 2003; Wang et al. 2004). The surprising theme that surfaced in these analyses was that all B-CLL cases displayed a common gene expression profile that is independent of the level of IgV gene somatic hypermutation (Klein et al. 2001; Rosenwald et al. 2001) or the expression of CD38 (Dürig et al. 2003). This finding implies that B-CLL represents a homogeneous disease despite genotypic (IgV gene mutational status and genomic alterations) and clinical differences. Unsupervised hierarchical clustering or supervised analysis of phenotypically or genotypically defined subgroups in the various studies generally yielded only a small number of gene expression differences (see Sect. 3). Overall, these observations did not support the hypothesis introduced above that B-CLL reflect distinct B cell developmental stages, as, for instance, is the case for diffuse large B cell lymphoma (DLBCL) (Alizadeh et al. 2000; Shipp et al. 2002). These observations, on the other hand, are consistent with the notion that all B-CLL derive from a common cellular precursor that has been subjected to a common pathogenetic mechanism (see Sect. 4).

B-CLL gene expression profiles have been compared against (1) age-matched, peripheral blood B cells (Jelinek et al. 2003), (2) normal B lymphocytes of different developmental stages, and (3) malignant B cells of other tumor types (Klein et al. 2001; Rosenwald et al. 2001). The B-CLL gene expression signatures identified in these studies were considerably overlapping despite using different microarray platforms (Klein et al. 2001; Rosenwald et al. 2001). A further analysis by Wang et al. compared the B-CLL microarray data from the previous studies with their own expression data using a different gene chip platform (Wang et al. 2004). Their results indicate that differences between the genes in the signatures are due to the variation in the representation of genes on the microarrays, rather than to methodological or technical differences attributed to the isolation procedures or the various platforms. Similarly, a work that compared B-CLL microarray data from different laboratories using the same platform (i.e., Affymetrix oligonucleotide arrays) found the data to be highly consistent (Jelinek et al. 2003). Thus, the B-CLL signature appears to be very strong and truly different from other lymphoma subtypes, and indeed, by now a large number of genes/gene products have been verified in independent panels by polymerase chain reaction (PCR) and Northern and Western blot analyses (Rosenwald et al. 2001; Jelinek et al. 2003; and our own unpublished data). Therefore, many of the B-CLL-specific genes identified by the gene expression profiling, including the protein tyrosine kinase ZAP-70 (see Sect. PackageErrorxmlreadUnknown crossref type seeheading) and the guanosine diphosphate (GDP) exchange factor EPAC (exchange protein activated by cyclic AMP) (Klein et al. 2001; Tiwari et al. 2004), are being studied and/or used for diagnostic purposes. Another observation from the B-CLL-specific signature was that the mRNAs encoding cell cycle-associated genes were downregulated compared to all normal and transformed B cells analyzed, even below levels of normal resting B cells (Klein et al. 2001). This finding is in accordance with the low proliferative capacity of the B-CLL tumor cells, although this type of analysis cannot exclude that a small fraction of cells may be proliferating and may not be abundant enough to confer a proliferative signature to the overall population (Chiorazzi and Ferrarini 2003).

Finally, the comparative analysis of the gene expression profiles of B-CLL with normal B cells (Klein et al. 2001; Rosenwald et al. 2001; Jelinek et al. 2003) yielded a large amount of new information to dissect the B-CLL phenotype. For instance, consistent with the known long-lived and apoptosis-resistant phenotype of B-CLL, pro-apoptotic genes were found to be downregulated and anti-apoptotic genes upregulated in the tumor cells. The upregulation of mRNA encoding several cytokine and chemokine receptors suggests that the tumor cells may react to certain stimuli abnormally compared to their normal counterparts. Clearly, the gene expression data obtained so far will prompt future studies on B-CLL and should eventually yield insights into its pathogenesis, and perhaps also identify suitable therapeutic targets.

3
B-CLL Subtypes

Perhaps the main objective of the initial microarray analyses was to identify genes whose expression is associated with a certain B-CLL subtype, defined through patient survival and disease staging (Stratowa et al. 2001), IgV mutational status (Klein et al. 2001; Rosenwald et al. 2001), or CD38-expression (Dürig et al. 2003). These approaches were meant to provide insights into the pathogenesis and derivation of the various subtypes, and the comparison of the IgV gene-mutated and -unmutated B-CLL cases was expected to provide clues about the derivation and the distinct clinical course of the subgroups. Although, as already pointed out in the previous section, IgV gene-mutated and -unmutated B-CLL cases do not separate in unsupervised hierarchical cluster analyses and exhibit a generally homogeneous gene expression profile (Klein et al. 2001; Rosenwald et al. 2001), supervised analysis of the two subgroups *did* identify a small set of genes that could be used to predict the IgV gene mutational status of B-CLL cases in independent panels (Klein et al. 2001; Rosenwald et al. 2001). This shows that although the gene expression differences between IgV-mutated and -unmutated B-CLLs are subtle, they reflect a consistent phenotypic difference between the subgroups.

Several studies investigated otherwise phenotypically (Dürig et al. 2003) or clinically (Stratowa et al. 2001) defined subtypes of B-CLL, or found evidence for subgroups among the analyzed B-CLL cases (Dürig et al. 2003; Jelinek et al. 2003). Thus, Dürig et al. aimed at identifying differences in the gene expression profile of CD38$^+$ and CD38$^-$ B-CLL cases and found only very few differences in gene expression (Dürig et al. 2003). The same study identified two subgroups of B-CLLs by unsupervised clustering within the same panel; one of those subgroups reportedly comprises patients with a more favorable clinical course with longer progression-free survival and reduced chemotherapy requirements (Dürig et al. 2003). Stratowa et al. report the identification of a set of genes whose expression levels correlated with patient survival and/or clinical staging (Stratowa et al. 2001). A third group, Jelinek et al., identified a small set of genes that may distinguish between low-risk (Rai stage 0) and high-risk (Rai stage 4) patients (Jelinek et al. 2003). We would like to note, however, that although all of these studies may identify a trend, the significance of the gene expression differences within the B-CLL panels reported in the above works remains uncertain. This is because the respective sets of genes discriminating potential B-CLL subtypes were not used to generate a classifier that can predict subtypes and were not validated in independent panels for their ability to classify. As an additional complication, in two of the quoted studies (Stratowa et al. 2001; Dürig et al. 2003), B-CLL cells were not purified. In our own experience, it was absolutely necessary to purify the tumor cells in order to identify gene expression differences among the IgV-mutated and -unmutated B-CLLs by supervised analysis. The specific signatures established on purified cells could then be used to interrogate and successfully classify unpurified samples (Klein et al. 2001; Rosenwald et al. 2001). We believe that cellular contamination of the peripheral blood samples drawn from B-CLL patients, even if highly enriched for tumor cells, has a profound impact on the analysis of unpurified tumor cells, because B-CLL cells seem to contain low levels of mRNA.

Do the IgV gene-mutated versus -unmutated gene expression profiles provide new information about those B-CLL subtypes? It has been noted that the IgV gene-unmutated tumor cells, in contrast to the mutated B-CLLs, express higher levels of genes that are activated during in vitro activation of B lymphocytes, leading to the suggestion that the IgV-unmutated B-CLL cells have ongoing B cell receptor (BCR) signaling (Rosenwald et al. 2001). Perhaps more relevant, ZAP-70, a member of the Syk-ZAP-70 protein tyrosine kinase family involved in T cell activation, was found to be specifically associated with the unmutated B-CLL subgroup (Rosenwald et al. 2001). On the one hand this finding will undoubtedly fuel new studies on BCR signaling in this B-CLL subtype; on the other it has already led to the development of flow-cytometric assays for the detection of ZAP-70, whose expression level may be used as a surrogate for the level of IgV gene mutational levels, and in turn predict the clinical course (Crespo et al. 2003; Orchard et al. 2004). However, while these analyses demonstrate a high level of concordance between IgV mutational status and ZAP-70 expression, the correlation is not absolute, suggesting that multiple determinants may be involved in the difference between the two subtypes of B-CLL.

Several studies comparing IgV gene mutation levels with IgV gene usage in B-CLL led to the conclusion that the expression of certain IgV gene segments correlates with their mutational status, and therefore also with clinical prognosis (this topic has been extensively reviewed by Chiorazzi and Ferrarini 2003). For example, certain V_H gene segments (e.g., *VH1-69*) occur generally in unmutated configurations, others (e.g., *VH3-07*) are strongly associated with IgV gene mutations (Chiorazzi and Ferrarini 2003). Contrary to those observations, a recent study showed that B-CLL cases that carry a rearranged *VH3-21* gene segment tend to have a poor overall survival independent of the level of IgV hypermutation (Tobin et al. 2003). In addition, these cases showed a restricted junctional repertoire, while the *VH3-21*-bearing heavy chain appeared to be predominantly associated with the expression of a particular λ light chain gene. Together, these observations, analogous to other V_H gene segments frequently observed in B-CLL (Chiorazzi and Ferrarini 2003), strongly imply a role for a common antigen in the development of *VH3-21*-bearing B-CLL cases. In turn, this implies that a B-CLL subtype can be defined by the expression of a particular V_H gene or V_H/V_L gene combination regardless of its IgV gene mutational level. Clearly, the results by Tobin et al. (2003) suggest a re-evaluation on the currently accepted subdivision of B-CLL cases: It may turn out that it is a particular antigen receptor that correlates with good or bad clinical prognosis, rather than the level of IgV somatic hypermutation in the rearranged V_H and V_L genes.

4 Cellular Derivation of B-CLL

B-CLL was long thought to be derived from the malignant transformation of $CD5^+$ B cells, which comprise a small subset of B cells in mice and humans. In favor of this hypothesis were observations made in mice that revealed that $CD5^+$ B cells have functional characteristics resembling B-CLL cells, such as long life, the capacity to replenish autonomously (Kantor et al. 1995), and the occasional ability to outgrow as a monoclonal population in old animals (Förster et al. 1988; LeMaoult et al. 1999). Others argued, however, that CD5 expression was merely a consequence of certain activation requirements, a notion supported by the observation that CD5 is upregulated by $CD5^-$ B cells upon in vitro stimulation (Wortis et al. 1995). $CD5^+$ B cells in mouse were long known to express a restricted antibody repertoire and to carry unmutated IgV genes (Kocks and Rajewsky 1989). In the human, $CD5^+$ B cells were analyzed by single-cell PCR (Brezinschek et al. 1997; Fischer et al. 1997; Geiger et al. 2000) (this approach became necessary as it avoids problems imposed by differing Ig mRNA levels among B cell subsets). These studies showed that the vast majority of $CD5^+$ B cells, across all ages, express unmutated IgV genes, thus mirroring the situation in the mouse. The actual IgV gene repertoire of human $CD5^+$ B cells, on the other hand, does not differ from that of $CD5^-$ B cells (Brezinschek et al. 1997). When it turned out that B-CLL can also express mutated IgV genes, models that invoked $CD5^+$ B cells as the precursors of B-CLL had to make the assumption that IgV-mutated B-CLL are derived from $CD5^+$ B cells that in rare instances proliferate and mutate their IgV genes in the GC reaction (Fischer et al. 1997). Meanwhile, putting more weight on the emerging picture that the IgV genes in unmutated B-CLLs show evidence of antigenic selection, alternative models of B-CLL pathogenesis were proposed (Oscier et al. 1997; Fais et al. 1998). These models referred to the canonical B cell developmental scheme, which states that B cells with unmutated IgV genes are naïve B cells, whereas somatically mutated B cells represent memory B cells, with the $CD5^+$ B cells being part of the naïve B cell fraction. However, an important, perhaps surprising element to resolve this controversy was provided by gene expression profile analysis, which basically ruled out the $CD5^+$ B cell as the principal normal counterpart of B-CLL since the gene expression profiles of B-CLL were vastly different from those derived from cord blood $CD5^+$ B cells (Klein et al. 2001; Rosenwald et al. 2001). Although it remains possible that $CD5^+$ B cells of newborns are different from age-matched $CD5^+$ B cells, overwhelming evidence (see below) suggested that $CD5^+$ B cells may not be related to B-CLL and thus may not represent the target of transformation in B-CLL.

Conversely, the comparison of the B-CLL gene expression data to B cell subset-specific signatures revealed that the gene expression profile of B-CLL, independent of the level of IgV gene mutation, was mostly related to that derived from tonsillar $CD27^+$ (memory) B cells (Klein et al. 2001). These observations led us to suggest that B-CLL may be derived from the malignant transformation of $CD27^+$ memory B cells (Klein et al. 2001). Nonetheless, several observations made over the last few years suggest that this $CD27^+$ fraction comprises a heterogeneous set of cells. First, and unexpected from the situation in the mouse, somatically mutated B cells in humans turned out to be surprisingly heterogeneous in their Ig isotype (Klein et al. 1998; Agematsu et al. 2000) and cell surface marker expression (Dono et al. 2000; Bar-Or et al. 2001), and also in terms of their function as suggested by in vitro studies (Agematsu et al. 1997; Kindler and Zubler 1997; Dono et al. 2001;

Werner-Favre et al. 2001). The apparent responsiveness of IgM-expressing CD27$^+$ B cells to T-independent antigens supported the suggestion that those cells might be marginal zone B cells (Dono et al. 2001; Werner-Favre et al. 2001), and thus the equivalent of murine marginal zone B cells, which are now generally accepted to comprise a separate B cell subset (Martin and Kearney 2002). Second, studies in the mouse showed that somatic hypermutation can occur outside the GC (William et al. 2002), and independent of T cells (de Vinuesa et al. 2000), although at significantly lower rates (Toellner et al. 2002); it has been proposed that also in the human, somatic hypermutation may be GC- and T-independent (Weller et al. 2001). Third, recent work on the peripheral B cell repertoire of either patients with genetic immune defects (Weller et al. 2004) or splenectomized children (Kruetzmann et al. 2003) brought up the intriguing possibility that the subset of somatically mutated IgM-expressing B cells is generated in an antigen-independent fashion, suggesting that somatic hypermutation can generate a diversified pre-immune repertoire, as is the case in sheep (Reynaud et al. 1995). IgM$^+$, IgV gene-mutated cells react to T-independent antigens and may be generated by a currently unknown extrafollicular pathway in the spleen (Kruetzmann et al. 2003; Weller et al. 2004).

Based on the above observations, it appears that mutated IgV genes and CD27-expression can be found in distinct B cell subpopulations and not only in post-GC memory B cells reacting to T-dependent antigens. (Of note, while unmutated IgV genes have been observed among CD27$^+$ cells, the reverse is almost never the case; CD27-negative B cells, which are generally IgM$^+$IgD$^+$, seem to be truly "naïve" in their Ig status.) Thus, it can be suggested that the CD27$^+$ population comprises "classical" memory B cells generated in the GC-reaction, antigen-experienced cells reacting to T-independent antigens, and perhaps a somatically mutated subset that may have been generated in a both antigen- and T-independent fashion. Because all of these cells can reside in the marginal zone of the peripheral lymphoid organs, one may collectively refer to them as marginal zone B cells. CD27$^+$ B cells of all isotype combinations (class switched, IgM-only, IgM$^+$IgD$^+$CD27$^+$) have indeed been shown to respond efficiently to various activation stimuli in vitro, while CD27$^-$ cells are less responsive or unresponsive (Agematsu et al. 1997; Kindler and Zubler 1997; Werner-Favre et al. 2001). Taken together, these observations suggest that while marginal zone B cells may represent developmentally distinct subsets, they may have the same function: to efficiently react to exogenous antigens and quickly differentiate into antibody-forming plasma cells.

The above-discussed features make marginal zone B cells, derived from either T-dependent or T-independent developmental stages, strong candidates for a normal counterpart of B-CLL. A large fraction of B-CLL expresses somatically mutated IgV genes, and CD27 is commonly expressed on the tumor cells (van Oers et al. 1993). While B-CLL cases are mainly $IgM^{+}IgD^{+}$, they can also be IgM only and class switched (Chiorazzi and Ferrarini 2003). The restricted IgV gene repertoire in both unmutated and mutated cases, as well as the evidence of antigenic selection in the mutated cases by R/S-values, suggests that antigen-stimulation plays a role at some point in B-CLL pathogenesis (discussed by Chiorazzi and Ferrarini 2003). Taken together, this evidence suggests that B-CLL predominantly originates through malignant transformation of marginal zone B cells (Fig. 1).

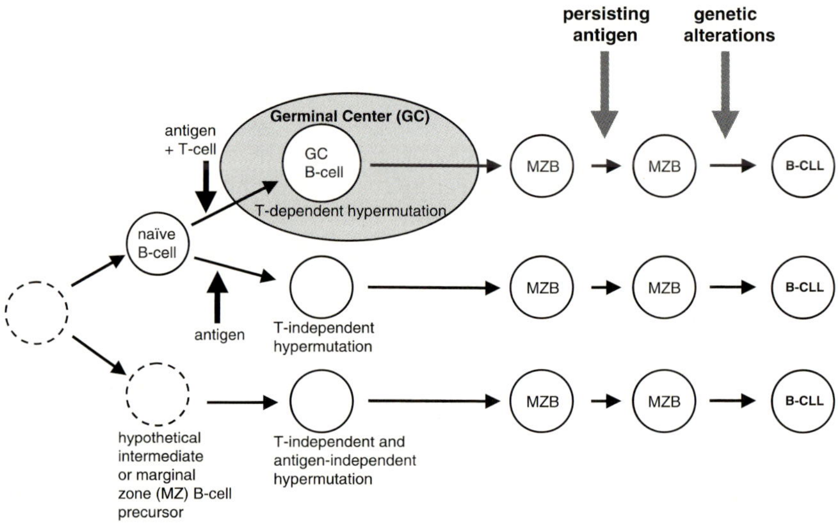

Fig. 1 A model for the cellular derivation of B-CLL. Antigen-inexperienced, naïve B cells may be driven into either a T-dependent or T-independent immune response (*top two branches*). A separate pathway (*bottom branch*) has been proposed recently in which somatically mutated B cells are generated in an antigen-independent fashion, suggesting that somatic hypermutation can generate a diversified pre-immune repertoire (see text). Upon completion of either the T-dependent GC response or the T-independent response(s), which may take place in a currently unknown extrafollicular pathway, the cells differentiate into marginal zone B cells (MZBs). MZBs may be continuously activated through persisting antigen and acquire genetic alterations that eventually lead to B-CLL development. *MZB*, marginal zone B cell; *GC*, germinal center

5 B-CLL Pathogenesis

The observation that B-CLL is more related to memory or marginal zone B cells than to any other known normal B cell subset suggests that the process leading to the clonal expansion may initiate in these cells. This notion is supported by the particular cytogenetic profile of B-CLL in relation to other B cell malignancies that are thought to originate from the malignant transformation of a GC-derived B cell. The GC-derived group of tumors, comprising e.g., DLBCL, follicular lymphoma (FL), Burkitt lymphoma (BL), and multiple myeloma (MM), are characterized by extensively mutated IgV genes and by the occurrence of specific reciprocal balanced chromosome translocations. Many of these translocations involve Ig loci, and the location of the breakpoints within the Ig loci suggest that the genomic alterations can be the result of mistakes in the recombination of the V, D, and J gene segments, Ig class switching, or IgV somatic hypermutation (reviewed by Küppers and Dalla-Favera 2001). The ongoing somatic hypermutation observed in FL and subsets of BL and DLBCL is suggestive of the tumor cells originating from a bona fide GC B cell. For the post-GC tumor MM, the malignant plasma cell equivalent, the discovery of pre-switch B cells clonally related to the MM cells suggested that the precursor cell preceding the MM clone might be a GC B cell (Corradini et al. 1993; Taylor et al. 2002). In contrast, despite showing IgV somatic mutations in a fraction of cases, B-CLL do not typically show reciprocal or other specific chromosome translocations (Döhner et al. 1999), although some exceptions have been reported (Döhner et al. 1999; Buhmann et al. 2002). Instead, the major genomic alterations are deletions and amplifications. This observation, together with the marginal zone B cell-like phenotype (see Sect. 4, above), suggests that B-CLL may lack chromosome translocations because the mechanisms involved in these aberrations, somatic hypermutation and Ig class switch, are no longer active in these cells (Fig. 2).

As to what may be the transforming mechanisms leading to B-CLL development, this is an open question and out of the scope of this review. Briefly, B-CLL is characterized by only a few common chromosome abnormalities including an association with 13q14 deletions that is present in around 50% of cases, depending on the panel studied (Corcoran et al. 1998; Döhner et al. 1999; Mabuchi et al. 2001; Migliazza et al. 2001). These deletions are thought to reflect the inactivation of an as-yet-unknown tumor-suppressor gene. Generally, the homogeneous gene expression profile of B-CLL suggests that its pathogenesis is associated with a largely common mechanism of transformation.

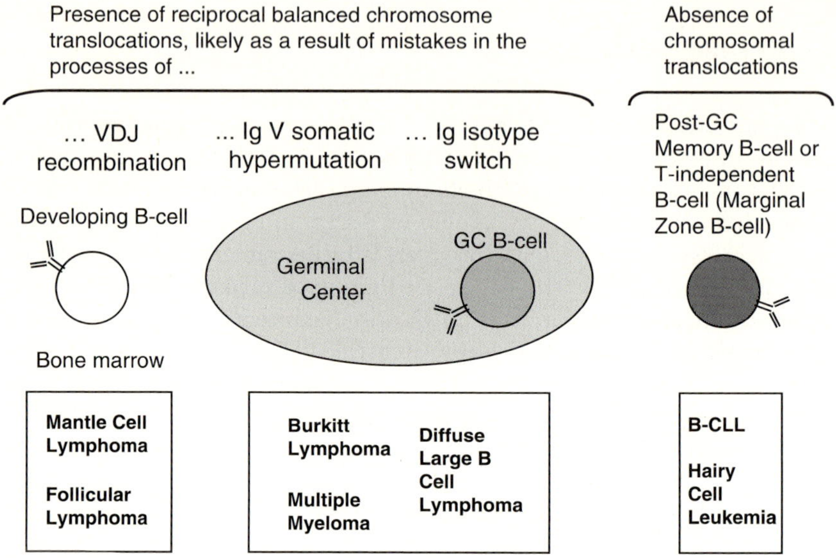

Fig. 2 Genetic aberrations and Ig-modifying processes. The major types of non-Hodgkin lymphoma, including mantle cell lymphoma, follicular lymphoma, Burkitt lymphoma, diffuse large B cell lymphoma, and multiple myeloma, are characterized by the presence of reciprocal balanced chromosome translocations that are likely a result of mistakes during VDJ recombination, IgV somatic hypermutation, or Ig isotype switch. On the other hand, B-CLL and hairy cell leukemia (HCL) lack such translocations, suggesting that the mechanisms involved in these aberrations are no longer active in the B-CLL and HCL precursor cells

A number of recent large-scale IgV gene repertoire analyses strongly imply the role for antigen in the development of B-CLL. Not only are particular IgV_H gene segments over-represented in antibodies expressed by B-CLLs (Chiorazzi and Ferrarini 2003), but there is also strong evidence for selection of particular IgV_H and light chain combinations (Ghiotto et al. 2004; Kolar and Capra 2004), and subgroups of B-CLL show similar CDRIII regions of light and/or heavy chains (Widhopf et al. 2004). These observations may suggest that the binding of specific antigen receptors to particular foreign antigens or autoantigens provides a continuous stimulatory signal through the BCR that keeps the B-CLL precursor in cell cycle for long periods of time and eventually allows for the acquisition of genomic aberrations.

Finally, we would like to introduce the possibility that B-CLL and hairy cell leukemia have a similar cell of origin. We have recently reported that HCL, whose phenotype is markedly distinct from B-CLL and any other lymphoma subtype (Harris et al. 1994), also resembles in its gene expression profile the $CD27^+$ B cells (HCL also expresses CD27) (Basso et al. 2004). As is the case for B-CLL, HCL lack chromosomal translocations (Haglund et al. 1994; Sambani et al. 2001). The fraction of cases expressing somatically mutated IgV genes, however, is higher in HCL compared to CLL (Maloum et al. 1998; Forconi et al. 2001). Perhaps B-CLL and HCL are commonly derived from the malignant transformation of a similar cellular precursor, a $CD27^+$ marginal zone or a memory B cell (Fig. 1). The different transformation processes acting on the precursor cells would determine their distinct phenotype and clinical presentation. Alternatively, the two tumor entities could be derived from the malignant transformation of distinct subsets of $CD27^+$ B cells (see previous section). In fact, a possible relationship between HCL and a particular tonsillar, somatically mutated B cell subpopulation (phab $V\text{-}3^+$, $CD27^+$, $CD11c^+$, $CD23^-$) has been noted (van Der Vuurst De Vries and Logtenberg 1999; Basso et al. 2004). Nonetheless, it might turn out that a subset of B cell malignancies including B-CLL and HCL is derived from a "group" of cells that was specifically generated for one purpose in immunity: to quickly establish an antibody-mediated immune response to foreign antigen.

6
Summary and Conclusions

Independent of their IgV gene mutational status, B-CLL cases resemble in their gene expression profile $CD27^+$ B cells, which represent a heterogeneous cell population with predominantly somatically mutated IgV genes, and mostly localize in the marginal zone or marginal zone equivalents. Clearly, the precise origin of B-CLL within this heterogeneous group of cells remains to be established. The identification of a subgroup of B-CLL cases with a particular V_H/V_L combination showing a generally unfavorable clinical course independent of the IgV mutational status suggests that the separation of B-CLL cases into IgV-unmutated and -mutated subgroups, and their association with good and bad prognosis, might have to be revised to include a critical role for the antigen. The absence in B-CLL of balanced reciprocal chromosome translocations that have been associated with mistakes in VDJ recombination, Ig class switching and somatic hypermutation suggest that the multistep transformation leading to B-CLL begins in a cell where these mechanisms are no longer active, consistent with a memory/marginal zone derivation. While global gene expression profile analysis has provided new insights into the phenotype and cell derivation of B-CLL, several gene products identified in those analyses might turn out to be targets for improved diagnosis and therapy. Unfortunately, the genetic alterations that are associated with the pathogenesis of this disease are still obscure.

Acknowledgements Research grants and other financial support: U.K. was the recipient of a fellowship granted by the Human Frontiers Science Program. This study has been supported by grants from the NIH (CA-37295) to R.D.-F.

References

Agematsu K, Nagumo H, Yang FC, Nakazawa T, Fukushima K, Ito S, Sugita K, Mori T, Kobata T, Morimoto C, Komiyama A (1997) B cell subpopulations separated by CD27 and crucial collaboration of CD27+ B cells and helper T cells in immunoglobulin production. Eur J Immunol 27:2073–2079

Agematsu K, Hokibara S, Nagumo H, Komiyama A (2000) CD27: a memory B-cell marker. Immunol Today 21:204–206

Alizadeh AA, Eisen MB, Davis RE, Ma C, Lossos IS, Rosenwald A, Boldrick JC, Sabet H, Tran T, Yu X, Powell JI, Yang L, Marti GE, Moore T, Hudson J Jr, Lu L, Lewis DB, Tibshirani R, Sherlock G, Chan WC, Greiner TC, Weisenburger DD, Armitage JO, Warnke R, Staudt LM, et al (2000) Distinct types of diffuse large B-cell lymphoma identified by gene expression profiling. Nature 403:503–511

Bar-Or A, Oliveira EM, Anderson DE, Krieger JI, Duddy M, O'Connor KC, Hafler DA (2001) Immunological memory: contribution of memory B cells expressing costimulatory molecules in the resting state. J Immunol 167:5669–5677

Basso K, Liso A, Tiacci E, Benedetti R, Pulsoni A, Foa R, Di Raimondo F, Ambrosetti A, Califano A, Klein U, Dalla-Favera R, Falini B (2004) Gene expression profiling of hairy cell leukemia reveals a phenotype related to memory B cells with altered expression of chemokine and adhesion receptors. J Exp Med 199:59–68

Brezinschek HP, Foster SJ, Brezinschek RI, Dorner T, Domiati-Saad R, Lipsky PE (1997) Analysis of the human VH gene repertoire. Differential effects of selection and somatic hypermutation on human peripheral CD5(+)/IgM+ and CD5(-)/IgM+ B cells. J Clin Invest 99:2488–2501

Buhmann R, Kurzeder C, Rehklau J, Westhaus D, Bursch S, Hiddemann W, Haferlach T, Hallek M, Schoch C (2002) CD40L stimulation enhances the ability of conventional metaphase cytogenetics to detect chromosome aberrations in B-cell chronic lymphocytic leukaemia cells. Br J Haematol 118:968–975

Caligaris-Cappio F, Hamblin TJ (1999) B-cell chronic lymphocytic leukemia: a bird of a different feather. J Clin Oncol 17:399–408

Chiorazzi N, Ferrarini M (2003) B cell chronic lymphocytic leukemia: lessons learned from studies of the B cell antigen receptor. Annu Rev Immunol 21:841–894

Corcoran MM, Rasool O, Liu Y, Iyengar A, Grander D, Ibbotson RE, Merup M, Wu X, Brodyansky V, Gardiner AC, Juliusson G, Chapman RM, Ivanova G, Tiller M, Gahrton G, Yankovsky N, Zabarovsky E, Oscier DG, Einhorn S (1998) Detailed molecular delineation of 13q14.3 loss in B-cell chronic lymphocytic leukemia. Blood 91:1382–1390

Corradini P, Boccadoro M, Voena C, Pileri A (1993) Evidence for a bone marrow B cell transcribing malignant plasma cell VDJ joined to C mu sequence in immunoglobulin (IgG)- and IgA-secreting multiple myelomas. J Exp Med 178:1091–1096

Crespo M, Bosch F, Villamor N, Bellosillo B, Colomer D, Rozman M, Marce S, Lopez-Guillermo A, Campo E, Montserrat E (2003) ZAP-70 expression as a surrogate for immunoglobulin-variable-region mutations in chronic lymphocytic leukemia. N Engl J Med 348:1764–1775

Damle RN, Wasil T, Fais F, Ghiotto F, Valetto A, Allen SL, Buchbinder A, Budman D, Dittmar K, Kolitz J, Lichtman SM, Schulman P, Vinciguerra VP, Rai KR, Ferrarini M, Chiorazzi N (1999) Ig V gene mutation status and CD38 expression as novel prognostic indicators in chronic lymphocytic leukemia. Blood 94:1840–1847

de Vinuesa CG, Cook MC, Ball J, Drew M, Sunners Y, Cascalho M, Wabl M, Klaus GG, MacLennan IC (2000) Germinal centers without T cells. J Exp Med 191:485–494

Dighiero G, Kipps T, Schroeder HW, Chiorazzi N, Stevenson F, Silberstein LE, Caligaris-Cappio F, Ferrarini M (1996) What is the CLL B-lymphocyte? Leuk Lymphoma 22 Suppl 2:13–39

Döhner H, Stilgenbauer S, Döhner K, Bentz M, Lichter P (1999) Chromosome aberrations in B-cell chronic lymphocytic leukemia: reassessment based on molecular cytogenetic analysis. J Mol Med 77:266–281

Dono M, Zupo S, Leanza N, Melioli G, Fogli M, Melagrana A, Chiorazzi N, Ferrarini M (2000) Heterogeneity of tonsillar subepithelial B lymphocytes, the splenic marginal zone equivalents. J Immunol 164:5596–5604

Dono M, Zupo S, Massara R, Ferrini S, Melagrana A, Chiorazzi N, Ferrarini M (2001) In vitro stimulation of human tonsillar subepithelial B cells: requirement for interaction with activated T cells. Eur J Immunol 31:752–756

Dürig J, Nückel H, Hüttmann A, Kruse E, Hölter T, Halfmeyer K, Führer A, Rudolph R, Kalhori N, Nusch A, Deaglio S, Malavasi F, Möröy T, Klein-Hitpass L, Dührsen U (2003) Expression of ribosomal and translation-associated genes is correlated with a favorable clinical course in chronic lymphocytic leukemia. Blood 101:2748–2755

Fais F, Ghiotto F, Hashimoto S, Sellars B, Valetto A, Allen SL, Schulman P, Vinciguerra VP, Rai K, Rassenti LZ, Kipps TJ, Dighiero G, Schroeder HW Jr, Ferrarini M, Chiorazzi N (1998) Chronic lymphocytic leukemia B cells express restricted sets of mutated and unmutated antigen receptors. J Clin Invest 102:1515–1525

Fischer M, Klein U, Küppers R (1997) Molecular single-cell analysis reveals that CD5-positive peripheral blood B cells in healthy humans are characterized by rearranged Vkappa genes lacking somatic mutation. J Clin Invest 100:1667–1676

Forconi F, Sahota SS, Raspadori D, Mockridge CI, Lauria F, Stevenson FK (2001) Tumor cells of hairy cell leukemia express multiple clonally related immunoglobulin isotypes via RNA splicing. Blood 98:1174–1181

Förster I, Gu H, Rajewsky K (1988) Germline antibody V regions as determinants of clonal persistence and malignant growth in the B cell compartment. Embo J 7:3693–3703

Geiger KD, Klein U, Bräuninger A, Berger S, Leder K, Rajewsky K, Hansmann ML, Küppers R (2000) CD5-positive B cells in healthy elderly humans are a polyclonal B cell population. Eur J Immunol 30:2918–2923

Ghiotto F, Fais F, Valetto A, Albesiano E, Hashimoto S, Dono M, Ikematsu H, Allen SL, Kolitz J, Rai KR, Nardini M, Tramontano A, Ferrarini M, Chiorazzi N (2004) Remarkably similar antigen receptors among a subset of patients with chronic lymphocytic leukemia. J Clin Invest 113:1008–1016

Haglund U, Juliusson G, Stellan B, Gahrton G (1994) Hairy cell leukemia is characterized by clonal chromosome abnormalities clustered to specific regions. Blood 83:2637–2645

Hamblin TJ, Davis Z, Gardiner A, Oscier DG, Stevenson FK (1999) Unmutated Ig V(H) genes are associated with a more aggressive form of chronic lymphocytic leukemia. Blood 94:1848–1854

Hamblin TJ, Orchard JA, Gardiner A, Oscier DG, Davis Z, Stevenson FK (2000) Immunoglobulin V genes and CD38 expression in CLL [letter]. Blood 95:2455–2457

Hamblin TJ, Orchard JA, Ibbotson RE, Davis Z, Thomas PW, Stevenson FK, Oscier DG (2002) CD38 expression and immunoglobulin variable region mutations are independent prognostic variables in chronic lymphocytic leukemia, but CD38 expression may vary during the course of the disease. Blood 99:1023–1029

Harris NL, Jaffe ES, Stein H, Banks PM, Chan JK, Cleary ML, Delsol G, De Wolf-Peeters C, Falini B, Gatter KC (1994) A revised European-American classification of lymphoid neoplasms: a proposal from the International Lymphoma Study Group. Blood 84:1361–1392

Jelinek DF, Tschumper RC, Geyer SM, Bone ND, Dewald GW, Hanson CA, Stenson MJ, Witzig TE, Tefferi A, Kay NE (2001) Analysis of clonal B-cell CD38 and immunoglobulin variable region sequence status in relation to clinical outcome for B-chronic lymphocytic leukaemia. Br J Haematol 115:854–861

Jelinek DF, Tschumper RC, Stolovitzky GA, Iturria SJ, Tu Y, Lepre J, Shah N, Kay NE (2003) Identification of a global gene expression signature of B-chronic lymphocytic leukemia. Mol Cancer Res 1:346–361

Kantor AB, Stall AM, Adams S, Watanabe K, Herzenberg LA (1995) De novo development and self-replenishment of B cells. Int Immunol 7:55–68

Kindler V, Zubler RH (1997) Memory, but not naive, peripheral blood B lymphocytes differentiate into Ig-secreting cells after CD40 ligation and costimulation with IL-4 and the differentiation factors IL-2, IL-10, and IL-3. J Immunol 159:2085–2090

Kipps TJ (1998) Chronic lymphocytic leukemia. Curr Opin Hematol 5:244–253

Klein U, Rajewsky K, Küppers R (1998) Human immunoglobulin (Ig)M+IgD+ peripheral blood B cells expressing the CD27 cell surface antigen carry somatically mutated variable region genes: CD27 as a general marker for somatically mutated (memory) B cells. J Exp Med 188:1679–1689

Klein U, Tu Y, Stolovitzky GA, Mattioli M, Cattoretti G, Husson H, Freedman A, Inghirami G, Cro L, Baldini L, Neri A, Califano A, Dalla-Favera R (2001) Gene expression profiling of B cell chronic lymphocytic leukemia reveals a homogeneous phenotype related to memory B cells. J Exp Med 194:1625–1638

Kocks C, Rajewsky K (1989) Stable expression and somatic hypermutation of antibody V regions in B-cell developmental pathways. Annu Rev Immunol 7:537–559

Kolar GR, Capra JD (2004) Ig V region restrictions in human chronic lymphocytic leukemia suggest some cases have a common origin. J Clin Invest 113:952–954

Kruetzmann S, Rosado MM, Weber H, Germing U, Tournilhac O, Peter HH, Berner R, Peters A, Boehm T, Plebani A, Quinti I, Carsetti R (2003) Human immunoglobulin M memory B cells controlling Streptococcus pneumoniae infections are generated in the spleen. J Exp Med 197:939–945

Küppers R, Dalla-Favera R (2001) Mechanisms of chromosomal translocations in B cell lymphomas. Oncogene 20:5580–5594

Küppers R, Klein U, Hansmann ML, Rajewsky K (1999) Cellular origin of human B-cell lymphomas. N Engl J Med 341:1520–1529

LeMaoult J, Manavalan JS, Dyall R, Szabo P, Nikolic-Zugic J, Weksler ME (1999) Cellular basis of B cell clonal populations in old mice. J Immunol 162:6384–6391

Mabuchi H, Fujii H, Calin G, Alder H, Negrini M, Rassenti L, Kipps TJ, Bullrich F, Croce CM (2001) Cloning and characterization of CLLD6, CLLD7, and CLLD8, novel candidate genes for leukemogenesis at chromosome 13q14, a region commonly deleted in B-cell chronic lymphocytic leukemia. Cancer Res 61:2870–2877

MacLennan IC (1994) Germinal centers. Annu Rev Immunol 12:117–139

Maloum K, Magnac C, Azgui Z, Cau C, Charlotte F, Binet JL, Merle-Beral H, Dighiero G (1998) VH gene expression in hairy cell leukaemia. Br J Haematol 101:171–178

Martin F, Kearney JF (2002) Marginal-zone B cells. Nat Rev Immunol 2:323–335

Migliazza A, Bosch F, Komatsu H, Cayanis E, Martinotti S, Toniato E, Guccione E, Qu X, Chien M, Murty VV, Gaidano G, Inghirami G, Zhang P, Fischer S, Kalachikov SM, Russo J, Edelman I, Efstratiadis A, Dalla-Favera R (2001) Nucleotide sequence, transcription map, and mutation analysis of the 13q14 chromosomal region deleted in B-cell chronic lymphocytic leukemia. Blood 97:2098–2104

Orchard JA, Ibbotson RE, Davis Z, Wiestner A, Rosenwald A, Thomas PW, Hamblin TJ, Staudt LM, Oscier DG (2004) ZAP-70 expression and prognosis in chronic lymphocytic leukaemia. Lancet 363:105–111

Oscier DG, Thompsett A, Zhu D, Stevenson FK (1997) Differential rates of somatic hypermutation in V(H) genes among subsets of chronic lymphocytic leukemia defined by chromosomal abnormalities. Blood 89:4153–4160

Rajewsky K (1996) Clonal selection and learning in the antibody system. Nature 381:751–758

Reynaud CA, Garcia C, Hein WR, Weill JC (1995) Hypermutation generating the sheep immunoglobulin repertoire is an antigen-independent process. Cell 80:115–125

Rosenwald A, Alizadeh AA, Widhopf G, Simon R, Davis RE, Yu X, Yang L, Pickeral OK, Rassenti LZ, Powell J, Botstein D, Byrd JC, Grever MR, Cheson BD, Chiorazzi N, Wilson WH, Kipps TJ, Brown PO, Staudt LM (2001) Relation of gene expression phenotype to immunoglobulin mutation genotype in B cell chronic lymphocytic leukemia. J Exp Med 194:1639–1647

Sambani C, Trafalis DT, Mitsoulis-Mentzikoff C, Poulakidas E, Makropoulos V, Pantelias GE, Mecucci C (2001) Clonal chromosome rearrangements in hairy cell leukemia: personal experience and review of literature. Cancer Genet Cytogenet 129:138–144

Schroeder HW Jr, Dighiero G (1994) The pathogenesis of chronic lymphocytic leukemia: analysis of the antibody repertoire. Immunol Today 15:288–294

Shipp MA, Ross KN, Tamayo P, Weng AP, Kutok JL, Aguiar RC, Gaasenbeek M, Angelo M, Reich M, Pinkus GS, Ray TS, Koval MA, Last KW, Norton A, Lister TA, Mesirov J, Neuberg DS, Lander ES, Aster JC, Golub TR (2002) Diffuse large B-cell lymphoma outcome prediction by gene-expression profiling and supervised machine learning. Nat Med 8:68–74

Stratowa C, Löffler G, Lichter P, Stilgenbauer S, Haberl P, Schweifer N, Döhner H, Wilgenbus KK (2001) CDNA microarray gene expression analysis of B-cell chronic lymphocytic leukemia proposes potential new prognostic markers involved in lymphocyte trafficking. Int J Cancer 91:474–480

Taylor BJ, Pittman JA, Seeberger K, Mant MJ, Reiman T, Belch AR, Pilarski LM (2002) Intraclonal homogeneity of clonotypic immunoglobulin M and diversity of non-clinical post-switch isotypes in multiple myeloma: insights into the evolution of the myeloma clone. Clin Cancer Res 8:502–513

Tiwari S, Felekkis K, Moon EY, Flies A, Sherr DH, Lerner A (2004) Among circulating hematopoietic cells, B-CLL uniquely expresses functional EPAC1, but EPAC1-mediated Rap1 activation does not account for PDE4 inhibitor-induced apoptosis. Blood 103:2661–2667

Tobin G, Thunberg U, Johnson A, Eriksson I, Soderberg O, Karlsson K, Merup M, Juliusson G, Vilpo J, Enblad G, Sundstrom C, Roos G, Rosenquist R (2003) Chronic lymphocytic leukemias utilizing the VH3–21 gene display highly restricted Vlambda2–14 gene use and homologous CDR3s: implicating recognition of a common antigen epitope. Blood 101:4952–4957

Toellner KM, Jenkinson WE, Taylor DR, Khan M, Sze DM, Sansom DM, Vinuesa CG, MacLennan IC (2002) Low-level hypermutation in T cell-independent germinal centers compared with high mutation rates associated with T cell-dependent germinal centers. J Exp Med 195:383–389

van Der Vuurst De Vries AR, Logtenberg T (1999) A phage antibody identifying an 80-kDa membrane glycoprotein exclusively expressed on a subpopulation of activated B cells and hairy cell leukemia B cells. Eur J Immunol 29:3898–3907

van Oers MH, Pals ST, Evers LM, van der Schoot CE, Koopman G, Bonfrer JM, Hintzen RQ, von dem Borne AE, van Lier RA (1993) Expression and release of CD27 in human B-cell malignancies. Blood 82:3430–3436

Wang J, Coombes KR, Highsmith WE, Keating MJ, Abruzzo LV (2004) Differences in gene expression between B-cell chronic lymphocytic leukemia and normal B cells: a meta-analysis of three microarray studies. Bioinformatics 20:3166–3178

Weller S, Faili A, Garcia C, Braun MC, Le Deist FF, de Saint Basile GG, Hermine O, Fischer A, Reynaud C, Weill J (2001) CD40-CD40L independent Ig gene hypermutation suggests a second B cell diversification pathway in humans. Proc Natl Acad Sci U S A 98:1166–1170

Weller S, Braun MC, Tan BK, Rosenwald A, Cordier C, Conley ME, Plebani A, Kumararatne DS, Bonnet D, Tournilhac O, Tchernia G, Steiniger B, Staudt LM, Casanova JL, Reynaud CA, Weill JC (2004) Human blood IgM "memory" B cells are circulating splenic marginal zone B cells harboring a pre-diversified immunoglobulin repertoire. Blood 104:3647–3654

Werner-Favre C, Bovia F, Schneider P, Holler N, Barnet M, Kindler V, Tschopp J, Zubler RH (2001) IgG subclass switch capacity is low in switched and in IgM-only, but high in IgD+IgM+, post-germinal center (CD27+) human B cells. Eur J Immunol 31:243–249

Widhopf IG, Rassenti LZ, Toy TL, Gribben JG, Wierda WG, Kipps TJ (2004) Chronic lymphocytic leukemia B cells of over one percent of patients express virtually identical immunoglobulins. Blood 104:2499–2504

William J, Euler C, Christensen S, Shlomchik MJ (2002) Evolution of autoantibody responses via somatic hypermutation outside of germinal centers. Science 297:2066–2070

Wortis HH, Teutsch M, Higer M, Zheng J, Parker DC (1995) B-cell activation by crosslinking of surface IgM or ligation of CD40 involves alternative signal pathways and results in different B-cell phenotypes. Proc Natl Acad Sci U S A 92:3348–3352

CTMI (2005) 294:51–70

Chronic Lymphocytic Leukemia: Molecular Genetics and Animal Models

Y. Pekarsky · G. A. Calin · R. Aqeilan · C. M. Croce (✉)

Comprehensive Cancer Center, Ohio State University, 410 W. 12th Ave., Columbus, OH 43210, USA
Carlo.Croce@osumc.edu

Abstract Chronic lymphocytic leukemia accounts for almost 30% of all adult leukemia cases in the United States and Western Europe. Although several common genomic abnormalities in CLL have been identified, mutational and functional analysis of corresponding genes so far have not proved their involvement in CLL. Our latest studies demonstrated functional involvement of Tcl1 oncoprotein and microRNA genes in the pathogenesis of CLL. Deregulated expression of Tcl1 in transgenic mice resulted in CLL. These CLL tumors showed abnormalities in expression of murine microRNA genes *mmu-mir-15a* and *mmu-mir-16-1*. Interestingly, human homologs of these genes, *mir-15a* and *mir-16-1*, located at the chromosome 13q14 are also deleted in human CLL samples. In this review we summarize and discuss these new developments. These recently emerged insights into the molecular mechanisms of CLL will allow for the development of new approaches to treat this disease.

1
Chromosomal Abnormalities in CLL

Chronic lymphocytic leukemia (CLL) accounts for almost 30% of all adult leukemia cases in the Western world (Sgambati et al. 2001). CLL patients can survive for a number of years showing relatively mild symptoms (Sgambati et al. 2001). Indeed, a significant proportion of cases of this disease are diagnosed incidentally. CLL lymphocytes are resting cells with morphologically mature appearance that usually do not show any spontaneous proliferation in vitro (Bullrich and Croce 2001; Sgambati et al. 2001). CLL cells also show a low level of surface immunoglobulins and display CD5 positivity (Sgambati et al. 2001). Since CLL occurs more commonly in people with at least one first-degree relative with CLL, familial aggregation of this disorder has been known for many years (Bullrich and Croce 2001). However, no CLL predisposition locus has been identified so far by linkage studies. Molecular genetic methods such as polymerase chain reaction (PCR) and fluorescence in situ hybridization (FISH) have significantly improved our understanding of molecular events and prognostic markers in CLL. Genomic aberrations are detected in over 80% of CLL cases. The common chromosomal abnormalities in CLL include 13q deletions, 11q and 7q deletions, trisomy 12 and 17p deletions (Dohner et al. 2000). The 13q14 deletion is the most common CLL aberration and is seen in 50% of all cases, whereas only 18%–20% of CLL cases do not show any chromosomal changes (Dohner et al. 2000). 13q14 deletions also occur in ~50% of mantle cell lymphoma, in 16%–40% of multiple myeloma, and in 60% of prostate cancers (Bullrich and Croce 2001; Sgambati et al. 2001), suggesting that one or more tumor suppressor genes at 13q14 are important for the initiation and/or progression of these diseases. Several groups have used positional cloning to identify the gene or genes targeted by the deletions. A region of more than 1 Mb has been fully sequenced and characterized (Bullrich et al. 2001; Migliazza et al. 2001). At least 13 genes located in the minimally homozygous deleted region (of about 300 kb) or very close (about 500 kb in the centromeric direction) have been cloned: *FAM10A4* (family with sequence similarity 10, member A4; Sossey-Alaoui et al. 2002), *DLEU7* (Hammarsund et al. 2004), *DLEU1* (deleted in lymphocytic leukemia, 1; Liu et al. 1997; Wolf et al. 2001), *DLEU2* (deleted in lymphocytic leukemia, 2; Liu et al. 1997), *mir-15a* and *mir-16-1* (microRNA genes 15a and 16-1; Calin et al. 2002), *KCNRG* (potassium channel regulator; Ivanov et al. 2003), *RFP2* (ret finger protein 2, *LEU5*; Kapanadze et al. 1998), *C13orf1* (chromosome 13 open reading frame 1, *CLLD6*; Mabuchi et al. 2001), *KPNA3* (karyopherin alpha 3, importin alpha 4; Kohler et al. 1997), *RCBTB1* (regulator of chromosome condensation, RCC1), BTB (POZ domain containing protein 1, *CLLD7*; Mabuchi

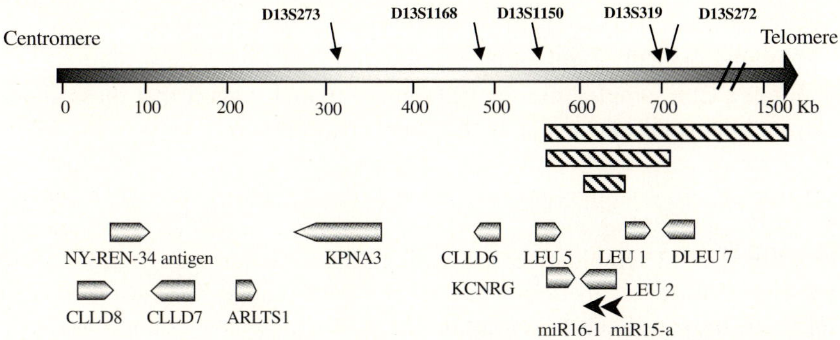

Fig. 1 Genomic organization of human chromosome 13q14 region. The exact position of the minimal regions of loss of heterozygosity (LOH) is presented as well as the position of all known genes in a region of ~1.5 Mb that was sequenced in our laboratory. *Diagonal striped bars* represent various LOH regions reported in the literature

et al. 2001), and *SETDB2* (SET domain, bifurcated 2, *CLLD8*; Mabuchi et al. 2001; Fig. 1). However, in spite of extensive research, none of the known genes of this region was found to be inactivated by a combination of deletion, mutation, or promoter hypermethylation (Bullrich et al. 2001; Migliazza et al. 2001; Rondeau et al. 2001; Mertens et al. 2002) as is proposed by the Knudson mechanism of inactivation of classical tumor suppressor genes (TSG).

In order to decipher the nature of elusive TSG at 13q14, in 2001 we generated somatic cell hybrids between mouse LMTK$^-$ and CLLs cells carrying 13q14 translocations and/or deletions and, using these hybrids identified a 30-kb region of deletion between exons 2 and 5 of the LEU2 gene (Calin et al. 2002). Since *LEU2* has been the subject of extensive study, and was excluded as a likely candidate tumor suppressor gene in CLL (Bullrich et al. 2001; Migliazza et al. 2001; Wolf et al. 2001; Mertens et al. 2002) we continued to search for genes within the region using publicly available sequence information and databases. This resulted in the discovery that a cluster of two noncoding microRNA genes, mir genes *mir-15a* and *mir-16-1*, is located precisely in the deleted region (Fig. 1; Calin et al. 2002).

The recent discoveries of the micro RNAs (miRNA) class of genes have taken the scientific community by storm, revealing a previously unknown layer of gene expression. The miRNAs are a large family of highly conserved non-coding genes thought to be involved in temporal and tissue-specific gene regulation (Storz 2002; Ambros 2004). miRNAs represent an evolving class of gene products with generally unknown function, and are usually excised from 60- to 70-nucleotide (nt) fold-back RNA precursor structures. Dicer RNase III and Argonaute family members are required for the miRNA precursor processing reaction (Hutvagner et al. 2001). The functional relevance of *mir-15a* and *mir-16-1* to CLL is still under investigation. However, our recent findings on human CLL samples and the CLL mouse model suggest that these genes play an important role in CLL pathogenesis (see Sect. 5).

2
CLL and Tcl1

2.1
TCL1 History and Genomic Organization

As mentioned above, although several common genomic abnormalities in CLL have been identified, mutational and functional analysis of corresponding genes so far did not prove their involvement in CLL. Generally, the final and conclusive proof for the involvement of any gene in any malignancy could be obtained only after studying transgenic and/or knockout animal models and showing symptoms of these malignancies in these models. Recently we have obtained such evidence for the *TCL1* oncogene in CLL (Bichi et al. 2002).

TCL1 oncogene was discovered as a target of inversions and translocations of *TCL1* (T cell leukemia/lymphoma 1) locus at 14q32.1, the most common chromosomal aberrations associated with mature T cell leukemias. Most often *TCL1* locus rearranges with the *TCR* (T cell receptor) α/δ locus at 14q11 (Russo et al. 1989; Virgilio et al. 1993). These rearrangements include inversion inv(14)(q11;q32) and translocation t(14;14) (q11;q32). Since both loci are located on the same chromosome, both of these rearrangements are reciprocal. In the case of the inversion inv(14)(q11;q32) the rearranged *TCL1* locus juxtaposed to the *TCR* α/δ receptor resulting in the abnormal chromosome 14. The translocation t(14;14) (q11;q32) results in the rearranged chromosome 14 containing two copies of the *TCL1* locus: the normal copy in the distal part of the chromosome and one rearranged copy in the proximity of the J segment of the *TCR* α/δ receptor. In both cases the *TCL1* locus juxtaposes to the regulatory elements of *TCR* α/δ receptor, therefore it seems possible that these elements are responsible for the activation of *TCL1* (Virgilio et al. 1994). Notably, inv(14)(q11;q32) and t(14;14) (q11;q32) were observed not only in patients with mature T cell leukemias but also in preleukemic conditions (Narducci et al. 1995; Thick et al. 1996), suggesting that rearrangements of the *TCL1* locus occur very early in the pathogenesis of mature T cell leukemia and that the activation of the *TCL1* locus is likely a causing event in the development of this disease.

Genomic mapping and characterization of breakpoint sequences within the *TCL1* locus revealed two breakpoint clusters separated by about 80 kb of DNA (Fig. 2; Virgilio et al. 1993) suggesting that genes targeted by the rearrangements at 14q32.1 are located within this 80-kb DNA segment. In 1994 we isolated the *TCL1* gene located in this breakpoint region breakpoint region (Virgilio et al. 1994). Several years later we completed characterization of the *TCL1* locus (Hallas et al. 1999; Pekarsky et al. 1999) and isolated three more genes. The *TCL1b* gene is located only 15 kb centromeric of *TCL1* with the opposite transcriptional orientation (Fig. 2; Pekarsky et al. 1999). The *TCL1* gene includes 4 exons and encodes a protein product of 114 amino acids (aa) (Virgilio et al. 1994). *TCL1b* also consists of 4 exons and encodes a larger Tcl1b polypeptide of 128 aa (Fig. 1). Interestingly, Tcl1b shows 60% similarity to Tcl1 at the amino acid level (Pekarsky et al. 1999). On the other hand, Tcl1 protein is also homologous to the Mtcp1 gene product. The *MTCP1* gene is located at Xq28 and activated in rare cases of mature T cell leukemia with a t(X;14)(q28;q11) translocation (Stern et al. 1993; Madani et al. 1996). Therefore the study of *TCL1* locus resulted in the identification of a new Tcl1 protein family containing three proteins: Tcl1, Tcl1b, and Mtcp1. Two other genes in the *TCL1* loci, *TNG1* and *TNG2* (*TCL1* neighboring genes 1 and 2), code for proteins not homologous to Tcl1 and are yet to be studied in detail.

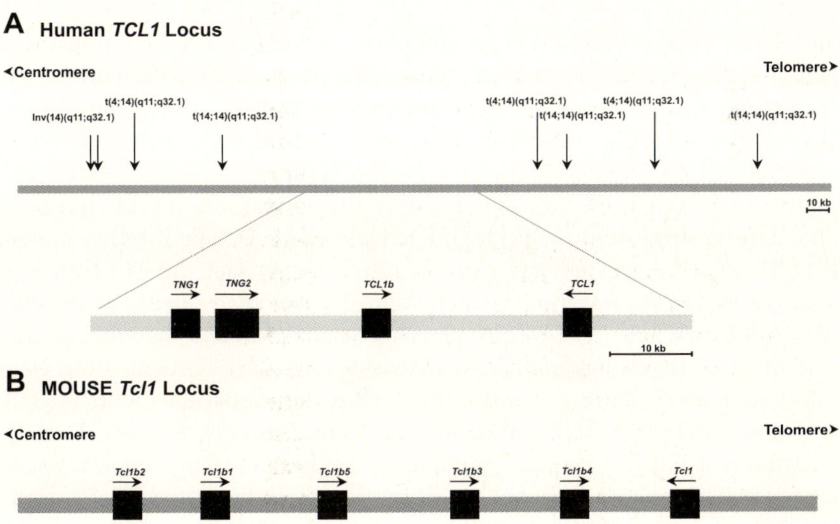

Fig. 2A, B Genomic organization of human and mouse *TCL1* locus. **A** Human locus; **B** Mouse locus. *Vertical arrows* represent positions of cloned 14q32.1 breakpoints from T-PLL/T-CLL

To isolate the mouse *Tcl1* gene family we studied the mouse *Tcl1* locus at chromosome 12 (Hallas et al. 1999). Sequence analysis of genomic clones within the locus resulted in the identification of a new and unexpected structure. The murine *Tcl1* locus contains six genes: one *Tcl1* gene and five *Tcl1b* genes (*Tcl1b1–5*) located within the 80-kb genomic locus (Fig. 3; Hallas et al. 1999). Our data suggest that murine *Tcl1b* encodes similar homologous proteins and all five genes express at least at the mRNA level. It is likely that these five genes were created by genomic duplication and it is not clear how many mouse Tcl1b proteins are functional.

The expression analysis of *TCL1* revealed the possible role of the protein in the development of leukemias and/or lymphomas (Virgilio et al. 1994). Tcl1 is expressed in the early stages of B cell development including early precursor (pre)-B cells, immunoglobulin (Ig)M-expressing cells and mantle cells, and, at lower levels, in germinal center B cells (Narducci et al. 2000; Said et al. 2001). On the other hand, Tcl1 expression is not detected in most mature B cells, i.e., plasma cells (Narducci et al. 2000; Said et al. 2001). Consequently almost all B cell lines (B-ALLs, Burkitt's lymphoma cells, and others) express Tcl1. Interestingly, Tcl1b shows a similar expression pattern at much lower levels, although the detailed study of its expression in B cell development is still lacking (Pekarsky et al. 1999). In contrast Tcl1 is not expressed in most T cells, except early $CD4^{-}$ $CD8^{-}$ T cells (Narducci et al. 2000). Non-lymphoid tissues and cell lines do not express Tcl1 (Virgilio et al. 1994). Notably, mouse *Tcl1* and *Tcl1b* show different expression patterns: the only expression of these genes is observed in eggs and very early embryonic stages, before blastocyst formation, and no significant presence is found in mouse lymphoid tissues (Hallas et al. 1999).

Since mature T cells do not express Tcl1 and the *TCL1* locus is rearranged in mature T cell leukemia, it is possible that inversions inv(14)(q11;q32) and translocations t(14;14) (q11;q32) activate *TCL1*. Detailed studies of mature T cell leukemia patients demonstrated that in fact the *TCL1* gene is a target of 14q32.1 rearrangements. Almost 100% of leukemia cases with inv(14)(q11;q32) or t(14;14) (q11;q32) show expression and therefore activation of *TCL1* (Brito-Babapulle and Catovsky 1991; Virgilio et al. 1994; Narducci et al. 2000). Even pre-leukemic T cell clones in patients with 14q32.1 rearrangements show Tcl1 expression (Narducci et al. 1995; Thick et al. 1996). Activation of Tcl1 has also been reported in acquired immunodeficiency syndrome (AIDS)-related immunoblastic lymphoma plasmacytoid (IBLP), a malignancy of mature B cell (Teitell et al. 1999). As mentioned above, mature B cells do not normally express Tcl1; in contrast, Tcl1 was detected in the majority of the AIDS IBLP samples (Teitell et al. 1999).

3
Tcl1 and Akt

3.1
Molecular Mechanisms

In the year 2000 we and others reported the involvement of *TCL1* in the *AKT (PKB)* oncogenic pathway (Laine et al. 2000; Pekarsky et al. 2000). Serine/threonine kinase Akt plays an important role in the regulation of signaling pathways involved in cell survival, proliferation, and death (Chan et al. 1999). A number of reports showed that Akt is an important molecule in determining the survival and proliferation of multiple cell types including B cells and T cells (Chan et al. 1999). Figure 3 shows the Akt signaling pathway. Growth and survival factors activate phosphatidylinositide 3-OH kinase (PI3K) in the plasma membrane (Chan et al. 1999). PI3K phosphorylates phospholipids located at the plasma membrane. Akt consists of two domains: pleckstrin homology (PH) domain and a kinase domain (Chan et al. 1999). PH domain is responsible for binding to phosphoinositides (PIP3) and protein–protein interactions; the kinase domain contains Thr308 and Ser473 residues important in the regulation of the enzymatic activity of Akt. Upon binding to phosphoinositides, Akt translocates to the plasma membrane where it gets phosphorylated at Thr308 and Ser473 and therefore activated (Fig. 3; Chan et al. 1999). This double-phosphorylated active Akt phosphorylates and regulates a number of pro- and anti-apoptotic factors including glycogen synthase kinase-3 (GSK3; Cross et al. 1995), IκB kinase-α (IKKα; Ozes et al. 1999), Bad (Bcl2 antagonist of cell death; Mok et al. 1999), cyclic AMP-responsive element binding protein (CREB; Du and Montminy 1998), and others.

Because of functional similarities of Tcl1 and Akt, we and others investigated whether these proteins might act in the same pathway (Laine et al. 2000; Pekarsky et al. 2000). Our results demonstrate that endogenous Akt and Tcl1 physically interact in lymphoid cells expressing both proteins (Pekarsky et al. 2000). Co-immunoprecipitation experiments also showed that exogenous Tcl1 and Akt physically interact in 293 and NIH-3T3 cells and the PH domain of Akt is responsible for this association (Pekarsky et al. 2000). What are the physiological consequences of this interaction? In vitro and in vivo kinase assay data revealed that Akt physically bound to Tcl1 shows significant increase in the kinase activity (Laine et al. 2000; Pekarsky et al. 2000) suggesting that Tcl1 functions as a co-activator of Akt. Since Akt is mostly cytoplasmic protein (Ahmed et al. 1993; Pekarsky et al. 2000) and Tcl1 is localized in both the cytoplasm and the nucleus (Narducci et al. 2000; Pekarsky et al. 2000), we investigated whether the Tcl1–Akt interaction affects

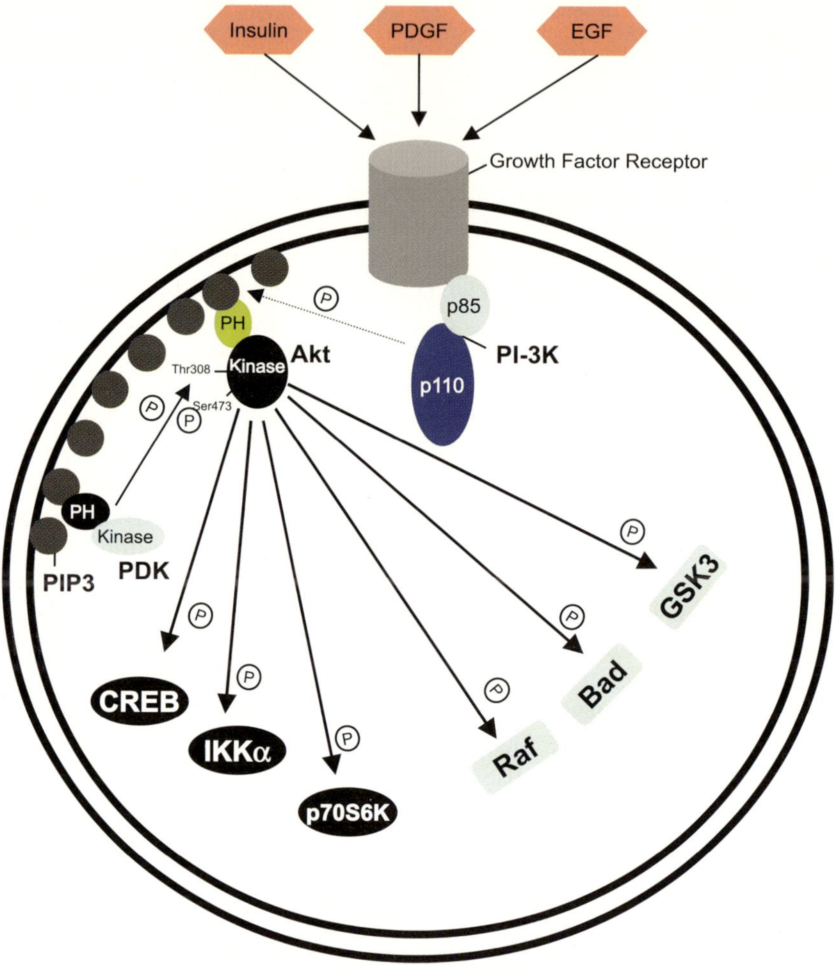

Fig. 3 Akt signaling pathway. Growth and survival factors activate PI-3 kinase (*PI3K*). PI3K phosphorylates phospholipids located at the plasma membrane. Akt consists of two domains: pleckstrin homology (*PH*) domain and a kinase domain. PH domain is responsible for binding to phosphoinositides (*PIP3*) and protein–protein interactions; the kinase domain is a catalytic domain and contains Thr308 and Ser473. Upon binding to phosphoinositides, Akt translocates to the plasma membrane where it gets phosphorylated by PDK1 at Thr308 and Ser473 and activated. This double-phosphorylated active Akt phosphorylates and regulates a number of pro- and anti-apoptotic factors. Activated targets are in *black* and inactivated targets are in *gray*

their intracellular location. Our immunofluorescence studies showed that Akt was co-expressed with Tcl1 located in both the cytoplasm and the nucleus. This suggests that Tcl1 mediates the nuclear translocation of Akt (Pekarsky et al. 2000). A recent report further investigated the role of dimerization and oligomerization of Tcl1 and Akt in the Tcl1–Akt interaction. Kunstle et al. demonstrated that mutations in Pro36, Leu37, and Thr38 of Tcl1 prevent its dimerization and that Asp16 and Ile74 of Tcl1 are important in the association of Tcl1 and Akt (Kunstle et al. 2002). Using different mutants of these residues, this study concluded that both dimerization of Tcl1 and physical binding to Akt are required for the full function of Tcl1 as an Akt kinase co-activator and for nuclear translocation of Akt mediated by Tcl1 (Kunstle et al. 2002).

As mentioned earlier in this section, a number of Akt targets were previously reported. It is important, therefore, to determine which of these downstream Akt targets is affected by Tcl1 expression as well as to identify Akt targets specifically expressed in lymphoid cells. In 2001 we and others identified the first known lymphoid-specific Akt target, Nur77 (Masuyama et al. 2001; Pekarsky et al. 2001). Nur77, also known as NGFI-B or TR3, is a member of the orphan nuclear receptor superfamily (Hazel et al. 1988). Nur77 is induced in T cells during TCR-mediated cell death (Liu et al. 1994), and this induction is required for apoptosis in T cell hybridomas and immature thymocytes (Calnan et al. 1995). Nur77 and two other members of this protein family, Nor1 and Nurr1 (Paulsen et al. 1995), are transcriptional activators. All three proteins contain DNA binding domains (DBD) and can bind DNA at specific *NGFI-B* response elements (NBRE) (Paulsen et al. 1995).

The DNA-binding ability of Nur77 is controlled in part by phosphorylation of Ser350 residue located within its DBD (Hirata et al. 1993; Katagiri et al. 1997). The residues surrounding Ser350 of Nur77 resemble the Akt phosphorylation consensus; therefore we (and others) investigated the possibility that Akt phosphorylates Nur77 at Ser350 (Masuyama et al. 2001; Pekarsky et al. 2001). Our data showed that Akt phosphorylates wild-type DBD of Nur77 in in vitro phosphorylation assays (Pekarsky et al. 2001). We further demonstrated that exogenously activated Akt phosphorylates Nur77 in 293 cells; and in NIH-3T3 cells, activation of endogenous Akt by PDGF resulted in phosphorylation of Nur77 at Ser350, and this phosphorylation was inhibited by Wortmannin, a PI-3 kinase (PI3K) inhibitor. Therefore, our results indicate that Akt phosphorylates Ser350 of Nur77 in a PI3K-dependent manner (Pekarsky et al. 2001). Since phosphorylation of Ser350 of Nur77 diminishes the DNA-binding ability of Nur77 (Hirata et al. 1993; Katagiri et al. 1997), we investigated whether phosphorylation of Nur77 by Akt causes similar effects. Using a luciferase assay system based on NBRE elements, we and others determined that this phosphorylation inhibits DNA-binding ability and transactivation ability of Nur77 by three- to sixfold (Masuyama et al. 2001; Pekarsky et al. 2001).

Figure 4 shows a schematic representation of the Tcl1-Akt-Nur77 pathway. Briefly, Tcl1 binds Akt, increases its kinase activity, and partially translocates Akt to the nucleus. Phosphorylation levels of the Akt targets increase, resulting in the increase of cell survival and resistance to apoptosis. In the case of Nur77, phosphorylation of Ser350 increases; therefore, the ability of Nur77 to bind DNA and to transactivate proapoptotic genes is diminished.

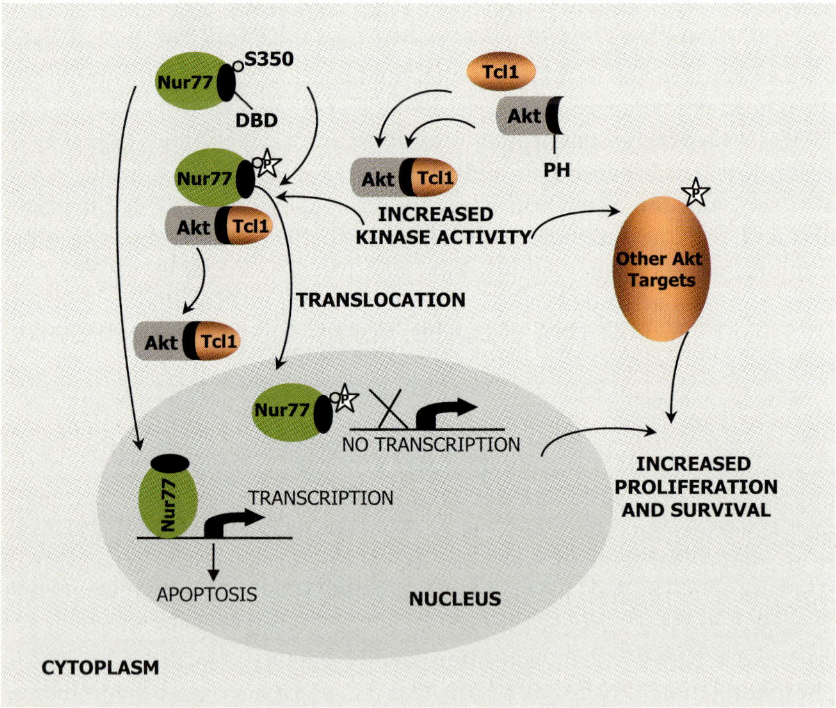

Fig. 4 Schematic representation of Tcl1-Akt-Nur77 pathway. Tcl1 binds Akt, increases its kinase activity, and partially translocates Akt to the nucleus. Phosphorylation levels of the Akt targets increase, resulting in the increase of cell survival and resistance to apoptosis. Normally Nur77 functions as a transcription factor, but, when phosphorylated by Akt, it cannot bind the DNA and is therefore inactive

4 Animal Models of CLL

Since expression of Tcl1 is detected at various levels in almost all stages of B cell development and is activated in AIDS IBLP, a B cell malignancy, it is possible that Tcl1 may also play a role in other B cell leukemias and lymphomas. To investigate this possibility, we and others recently created transgenic mouse models showing deregulated expression of Tcl1 in B cells (Bichi et al. 2002; Hoyer et al. 2002). We generated a transgenic mouse line expressing the human *TCL1* gene under the control of a V_H promoter Ig_H-Eμ enhancer to target transgene expression to immature and mature B cells (Bichi et al. 2002). At the age of 10–18 months these transgenic animals became visibly sick. Pathological analysis revealed enlarged liver and spleen and high white blood cell counts, on average 180×10^6 cells/ml compared with 2.8×10^6 cells/ml in wild-type animals (Bichi et al. 2002). The predominant leukemic cell type was represented in large lymph nodes and enlarged spleen. Histological analysis also revealed infiltration in lymph nodes, liver, and spleen by malignant lymphocytes; these cells as expected were human Tcl1 positive (Bichi et al. 2002). Flow cytometric analysis showed that these leukemic cells were CD5 and IgM positive, suggesting that these mice developed mature B cell leukemia, a disease very similar to human B-CLL (Bichi et al. 2002). A significantly enhanced $CD5^+$ cell population in the peritoneal cavity of these transgenic animals was observed by the age of 2 months, in spleen by the age of 3 to 5 months, and in bone marrow by the age of 5 to 8 months. Southern analysis of immunoglobulin gene rearrangements revealed the presence of pre-leukemic and leukemic clones, confirming the resemblance to human B-CLL (Bichi et al. 2002).

In the second report, Hoyer et al. described a *TCL1* transgenic mouse with the expression of *TCL1* in both B cells and T cells (Hoyer et al. 2002). These *TCL1* transgenic animals showed a phenotype very similar to that described in our report: at the average age of 12 months these mice became visibly sick with the accumulation of malignant B cells (Hoyer et al. 2002). In addition, these malignant B cells showed increased proliferation in vitro and increased survival in tissue culture experiments compared to splenic cells of wild-type mice (Hoyer et al. 2002).

These results suggest that deregulated expression of Tcl1 causes the development of B-CLL. Since Tcl1 is the Akt co-activator, it is likely that enhanced kinase activity of Akt is an important factor in the CLL pathogenesis. This also suggests that in order to uncover molecular mechanisms of CLL we need to determine which Akt targets' phosphorylation is affected by the deregulation of Tcl1 expression.

A very recent report described another transgenic mouse model for CLL. Planelles et al. reported that mice showing deregulated expression of APRIL (an acronym derived from a proliferation-inducing ligand) develop mature B cell leukemia resembling CLL at the age of 9–12 months (Planelles et al. 2004). APRIL is a secreted protein, a tumor necrosis factor (TNF)-like ligand, capable of stimulating tumor cell proliferation in vitro (Planelles et al. 2004). APRIL transgenic mice express this protein in T cells, causing elevated APRIL serum levels. Therefore, APRIL works systemically in these mice, affecting B cell survival. APRIL transgenic mice develop lymph node hyperplasia at the age of 9 months. Flow cytometric analysis showed that dramatically expanded B cells are $CD5^+$ and similar to CLL leukemic cells described above for *TCL1* transgenics (Planelles et al. 2004). Interestingly, APRIL was also overexpressed in a large fraction of B-CLL tumors, causing increased serum levels in B-CLL patients (Planelles et al. 2004). It is possible therefore that APRIL is a new important player in B-CLL pathogenesis, although the exact molecular mechanism of its function is not known.

5 The MicroRNAs in CLL: New Players in an Old Disease

The expectation was that the study of genomic alterations of the *TCL1* transgenic mice will highlight the important pathogenic abnormalities yet unknown or only partially deciphered. Analyzing the chromosomal constitution of blood, spleen, and bone marrow cells of the *TCL1* transgenic mice we found that the equivalents of the two most frequent human CLL chromosomal alterations were present: partial deletion of the long arm of chromosome 14 (the mouse homolog of human chromosome 13) as well as tri- and tetrasomy 15 (the mouse homolog of the human chromosome 12). Further refining the genomic dissection by using comparative genomic hybridization (CGH) showed deletions of a region of mouse chromosome 14 (of about 30 Mb) including, at the centromeric end, two microRNA genes, *mmu-mir-15a* and *mmu-mir-16-1* (Fig. 1). Interestingly, these are the mouse homologs of human *mir-15a* and *mir-16-1*, located at the chromosome region 13q14, deleted heterozygously in more than half and homozygously in about 10% of B-CLL cases. The cluster *mir-15a/mir-16-1* is located within a small deleted region (~30 kb) and is also involved in translocation in B-CLL, and both genes are deleted or downregulated in approximately 66% of CLL cases as compared with $CD5^+$ cells from healthy donors (Calin et al. 2002).

On the converse to the active transcription of all retained genes from the minimally LOH region, the miRNAs showed variations of expression correlated with the genomic status of the region (Fig. 5). For example, *DLEU 1* and *RFP5* show the same levels of expression in deleted versus non-deleted cases, indicating that the retained allele is apparently normally expressed, while *DLEU2* showed no detectable expression in B-CLL samples, regardless the 13q14.3 status (Bullrich et al. 2001; Migliazza et al. 2001). The two miRNAs located in this region show an expression correlated with the number of alleles present on the genome; furthermore, in several cases with both alleles normal, the expression is reduced. Therefore, it might be possible that epigenetic mechanisms (such as promoter methylation) are involved in silencing this new type of gene (Calin et al. 2002).

Mutation analysis in the exon coding genes from 13q13.4 failed to identify any pathogenetic mutation (Bullrich et al. 2001; Mabuchi et al. 2001; Migliazza et al. 2001; Calin et al. 2002). Using more sensitive expression analysis by quantitative reverse transcriptase (RT)-PCR of genes at 13q14.3, *RB1*, *CLLD7*, *KPNA3*, *CLLD6*, and *RFP2* were found downregulated in B-CLL patients as compared with B cells from healthy donors (Mertens et al. 2002). However, this tumor-specific phenomenon could not be associated with DNA methylation, because no difference in the methylation status was detected in any CpG island of the minimally deleted region (Mertens et al. 2002). Very recently, we have found mutations in the precursor of *mir-16-1* associated with malfunction of

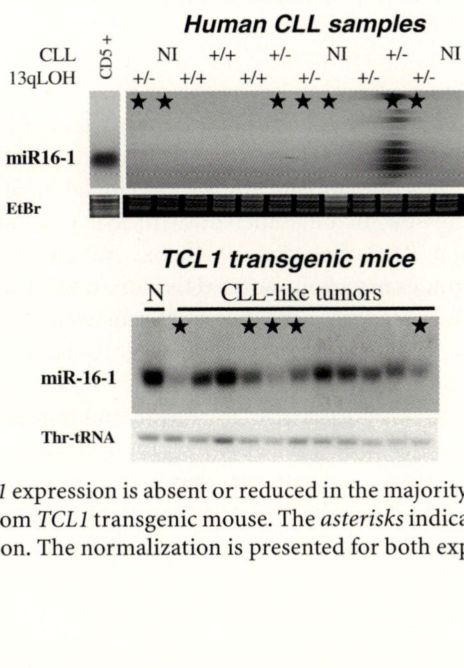

Fig. 5 *miRNA-16-1* expression is absent or reduced in the majority of human CLL and CLL-like tumors from *TCL1* transgenic mouse. The *asterisks* indicate the samples with abnormal expression. The normalization is presented for both experiments

the precursor processing (G. Calin and C.M. Croce, submitted manuscript). In all cases harboring mutations we have found LOH at 13q14, suggesting that the classical inactivation mechanism of a TSG (LOH+mutation) is valid also for microRNAs.

To further investigate the possible involvement of miRNAs on a genome-wide basis in CLL and in human cancers generally, we have mapped 186 miRNAs and compared their location to the location of previously reported non-random genetic alterations. We found that 98 of 186 (52.5%) known miRNA genes are frequently located at fragile sites, as well as in minimal regions of loss of heterozygosity (minimal LOH), minimal regions of amplification (minimal amplicons), or common breakpoint regions (Calin et al. 2004a). Much more significantly, a cluster of two microRNAs, *mir-34b* and *mir-34c*, is located in the region of 11q23, which is frequently deleted in human CLL and several other hematopoietic and solid cancers (Calin et al. 2000). By Northern blotting we have shown that several miRNAs found in deleted regions have low levels of expression in cancer samples (Calin et al. 2004a). These data provide a catalogue of miRNA genes (e.g., *mir-15a*, *mir-16-1*, *mir-34b* and *mir-34c*) that may have roles in human CLL and support the argument that the miRNome (defined as the full complement of miRNAs in a genome) may be extensively involved in this particular type of cancer.

6
MicroRNA Gene Expression Profiles in Normal Cells and Malignant CLL Cells Are Different

Assessing cancer-specific expression levels for hundreds of miRNA genes is time consuming, and requires a large amount of total RNA. Therefore, to overcome these limitations and investigate alterations in the expression of all known miRNAs in human cancers, we developed a miRNA microarray containing 368 gene-specific oligonucleotide probes generated from 161 human and 84 mouse miRNAs (Liu et al. 2004). First, we analyzed the microRNA gene expression profiles in various normal tissues; in unsupervised hierarchical clustering, we found that the same types of tissue from different individuals clustered together. The hematopoietic tissues aggregate in two distinct clusters, the first one contains $CD5^+$ cells, T lymphocytes, and leucocytes and the second cluster includes bone marrow, fetal liver, and B lymphocytes.

Second, we investigated the microRNA expression in $CD5^+$ cells from normal individuals and from CLL cells and identified a set of genes differentially expressed between the two types of cells. The list includes several miRNAs located exactly inside fragile sites (*mir-183* at FRA7H, *mir-190* at FRA12A and *mir-24-1* at FRA9D) as well as *mir-213*, expressed at lower levels in all analyzed CLL samples. *mir-16-1* and *mir-15a*, at 13q14.3, which we previously reported to be down-regulated in the majority of CLL cases by Northern blot analysis (Calin et al. 2002), were found to be expressed at low levels in 45% and ~25% of CLL samples, respectively, validating, therefore, the microarray data (Calin et al. 2004a). Overall, these data demonstrate that CLL is a malignancy with extensive alterations of miRNA expression and suggest a role for distinct miRNAs in the pathogenesis of human B cell malignancies.

Third, we asked if microarray data revealed specific molecular signatures predictive for subsets of CLL that differ in clinical behavior. It is well known that CLL patients with chromosome 13q14 deletions have a relatively good prognosis, compared with patients with leukemia cells harboring complex cytogenetic changes (Dohner et al. 2000). Furthermore, deletion at 13q14.3 was associated with the presence of mutated IgV_H genes (Oscier et al. 2002), another good prognostic factor. By comparing expression data of CLL samples with or without deletions at 13q14, we found that *mir-16-1* was expressed at statistically significant lower levels in leukemias harboring deletions at 13q14. We also found that *mir-24-2, mir-195, mir-203, mir-220*, and *mir-221* are expressed at significantly reduced levels in the samples with 13q14.3 deletions. Conversely, *mir-7-1*, *mir-19a*, *mir-136*, *mir-154*, and *mir-217* are expressed at significantly higher levels.

The expression of mutated IgV_H is a favorable prognostic marker in CLL (Dohner et al. 2000). We found a specific signature profile composed of five differentially expressed genes (*mir-186*, *mir-132*, *mir-16-1*, *mir-102*, and *mir-29c*) that distinguish CLL samples that expressed mutated IgV_H gene from those that expressed unmutated IgV_H genes, suggesting that miRNA expression profiles have prognostic significance in CLL. As a confirmation of our results is the observation that the common element between the del 13q14.3-related and the IgV_H-related signatures is *mir-16-1*. This gene is located in the common deleted region 13q14.3, and the presence of this particular deletion is associated with good prognosis. Therefore, miRNAs may expand the spectrum of adverse prognostic markers in CLL, such as the expression of ZAP-70, unmutated IgV_H, CD38, deletion at chromosome 11q23, or loss or mutation of *TP53* (Calin et al. 2004b).

7
Conclusions

Although several recurring chromosomal rearrangements in CLL have been studied in detail, only recently has this information started to provide clues of exact molecular mechanisms of the pathogenesis of this common leukemia. The Tcl1-Akt oncogenic pathway is the only proven functional insight into CLL pathogenesis, but the importance of this pathway needs to be further evaluated. Although *TCL1* was first discovered as an oncogene involved in mature T cell leukemias, several important studies significantly expanded the importance of this gene to a variety of leukemias and lymphomas including CLL. Reports showing that Tcl1 is a co-activator of Akt shed some light into the function of this protein. On the other hand, it is not clear whether involvement in the Akt pathway is the only function of Tcl1 or whether other, maybe even more important and interesting, molecular functions of Tcl1 exist. Clearly, better understanding of Tcl1 function is necessary in order to develop specific therapies for leukemias/lymphomas including CLL caused by *TCL1* deregulation.

Detailed genetic studies of deleted regions in CLL samples also revealed an unexpected finding: the involvement of a new class of genes, the microRNAs, as cancer players. We hypothesize that miRNAs could be contributors of oncogenesis working as classical TSG (as is the case of *mir-15a* and *mir-16-1*) or as classical oncogenes. The distinct expression of several miRNAs between normal and malignant cells, the presence of mutations as well as the possible differences in epigenetic regulation of miRNA expression argue that the full complement of miRNAs in a genome may be involved in cancer. The B-CLL is only the first histotype in which the microRNA gene alterations were dissected at the genomic level. Furthermore, because of the clear correlation with prognostic factors such as ZAP-70 or IgVH expression, miRNA expression may expand the spectrum of prognostic markers in CLL.

References

Ahmed NN, Franke TF, Bellacosa A, Datta K, Gonzalez-Portal ME, Taguchi T, Testa JR, Tsichlis PN (1993) The proteins encoded by c-akt and v-akt differ in post-translational modification, subcellular localization and oncogenic potential. Oncogene 8:1957–1963

Ambros V (2004) The functions of animal microRNAs. Nature 431:350–355

Bichi R, Shinton SA, Martin ES, Koval A, Calin GA, Cesari R, Russo G, Hardy RR, Croce CM (2002) Human chronic lymphocytic leukemia modeled in mouse by targeted TCL1 expression. Proc Natl Acad Sci U S A 99:6955–6960

Brito-Babapulle V, Catovsky D (1991) Inversions and tandem translocations involving chromosome 14q11 and 14q32 in T-prolymphocytic leukemia and T-cell leukemias in patients with ataxia telangiectasia. Cancer Genet Cytogenet 55:1–9

Bullrich F, Croce C (2001) Molecular biology of chronic lymphocytic leukemia. In: Bruce Cheson (ed) Chronic lymphocytic leukemias, 2nd edn, revised and expanded. Marcel Dekker, New York, pp 9–32

Bullrich F, Fujii H, Calin G, Mabuchi H, Negrini M, Pekarsky Y, Rassenti L, Alder H, Reed JC, Keating MJ, Kipps TJ, Croce CM (2001) Characterization of the 13q14 tumor suppressor locus in CLL: identification of ALT1, an alternative splice variant of the LEU2 gene. Cancer Res 61:6640–6648

Calin GA, di Iasio MG, Caprini E, Vorechovsky I, Natali PG, Sozzi G, Croce CM, Barbanti-Brodano G, Russo G, Negrini M (2000) Low frequency of alterations of the alpha (PPP2R1A) and beta (PPP2R1B) isoforms of the subunit A of the serine-threonine phosphatase 2A in human neoplasms. Oncogene 19:1191–1195

Calin GA, Dumitru CD, Shimizu M, Bichi R, Zupo S, Noch E, Aldler H, Rattan S, Keating M, Rai K, Rassenti L, Kipps T, Negrini M, Bullrich F, Croce CM (2002) Frequent deletions and down-regulation of micro-RNA genes miR15 and miR16 at 13q14 in chronic lymphocytic leukemia. Proc Natl Acad Sci U S A 99:15524–15529

Calin GA, Liu CG, Sevignani C, Ferracin M, Felli N, Dumitru CD, Shimizu M, Cimmino A, Zupo S, Dono M, Dell'Aquila ML, Alder H, Rassenti L, Kipps TJ, Bullrich F, Negrini M, Croce CM (2004a) MicroRNA profiling reveals distinct signatures in B cell chronic lymphocytic leukemias. Proc Natl Acad Sci U S A 101:11755–11760

Calin GA, Sevignani C, Dumitru CD, Hyslop T, Noch E, Yendamuri S, Shimizu M, Rattan S, Bullrich F, Negrini M, Croce CM (2004b) Human microRNA genes are frequently located at fragile sites and genomic regions involved in cancers. Proc Natl Acad Sci U S A 101:2999–3004

Calnan BJ, Szychowski S, Chan FK, Cado D, Winoto A (1995) A role for the orphan steroid receptor Nur77 in apoptosis accompanying antigen-induced negative selection. Immunity 3:273–282

Chan TO, Rittenhouse SE, Tsichlis PN (1999) AKT/PKB and other D3 phosphoinositide-regulated kinases: kinase activation by phosphoinositide-dependent phosphorylation. Annu Rev Biochem 68:965–1014

Cross DA, Alessi DR, Cohen P, Andjelkovich M, Hemmings BA (1995) Inhibition of glycogen synthase kinase-3 by insulin mediated by protein kinase B. Nature 378:785–789

Dohner H, Stilgenbauer S, Benner A, Leupolt E, Krober A, Bullinger L, Dohner K, Bentz M, Lichter P (2000) Genomic aberrations and survival in chronic lymphocytic leukemia. N Engl J Med 343:1910–1916

Du K, Montminy M (1998) CREB is a regulatory target for the protein kinase Akt/PKB. J Biol Chem 273:32377–32379

Hallas C, Pekarsky Y, Itoyama T, Varnum J, Bichi R, Rothstein JL, Croce CM (1999) Genomic analysis of human and mouse TCL1 loci reveals a complex of tightly clustered genes. Proc Natl Acad Sci U S A 96:14418–14423

Hammarsund M, Corcoran MM, Wilson W, Zhu C, Einhorn S, Sangfelt O, Grander D (2004) Characterization of a novel B-CLL candidate gene—DLEU7—located in the 13q14 tumor suppressor locus. FEBS Lett 556:75–80

Hazel TG, Nathans D, Lau LF (1988) A gene inducible by serum growth factors encodes a member of the steroid and thyroid hormone receptor superfamily. Proc Natl Acad Sci U S A 85:8444–8448

Hirata Y, Kiuchi K, Chen HC, Milbrandt J, Guroff G (1993) The phosphorylation and DNA binding of the DNA-binding domain of the orphan nuclear receptor NGFI-B. J Biol Chem 268:24808–24812

Hoyer KK, French SW, Turner DE, Nguyen MT, Renard M, Malone CS, Knoetig S, Qi CF, Su TT, Cheroutre H, Wall R, Rawlings DJ, Morse HC 3rd, Teitell MA (2002) Dysregulated TCL1 promotes multiple classes of mature B cell lymphoma. Proc Natl Acad Sci U S A 99:14392–14397

Hutvagner G, McLachlan J, Pasquinelli AE, Balint E, Tuschl T, Zamore PD (2001) A cellular function for the RNA-interference enzyme Dicer in the maturation of the let-7 small temporal RNA. Science 293:834–838

Ivanov DV, Tyazhelova TV, Lemonnier L, Kononenko N, Pestova AA, Nikitin EA, Prevarskaya N, Skryma R, Panchin YV, Yankovsky NK, Baranova AV (2003) A new human gene KCNRG encoding potassium channel regulating protein is a cancer suppressor gene candidate located in 13q14.3. FEBS Lett 539:156–160

Kapanadze B, Kashuba V, Baranova A, Rasool O, van Everdink W, Liu Y, Syomov A, Corcoran M, Poltaraus A, Brodyansky V, Syomova N, Kazakov A, Ibbotson R, van den Berg A, Gizatullin R, Fedorova L, Sulimova G, Zelenin A, Deaven L, Lehrach H, Grander D, Buys C, Oscier D, Zabarovsky ER, Yankovsky N (1998) A cosmid and cDNA fine physical map of a human chromosome 13q14 region frequently lost in B-cell chronic lymphocytic leukemia and identification of a new putative tumor suppressor gene, Leu5. FEBS Lett 426:266–270

Katagiri Y, Hirata Y, Milbrandt J, Guroff G (1997) Differential regulation of the transcriptional activity of the orphan nuclear receptor NGFI-B by membrane depolarization and nerve growth factor. J Biol Chem 272:31278–31284

Kohler M, Ansieau S, Prehn S, Leutz A, Haller H, Hartmann E (1997) Cloning of two novel human importin-alpha subunits and analysis of the expression pattern of the importin-alpha protein family. FEBS Lett 417:104–108

Kunstle G, Laine J, Pierron G, Kagami Si S, Nakajima H, Hoh F, Roumestand C, Stern MH, Noguchi M (2002) Identification of Akt association and oligomerization domains of the Akt kinase coactivator TCL1. Mol Cell Biol 22:1513–1525

Laine J, Kunstle G, Obata T, Sha M, Noguchi M (2000) The protooncogene TCL1 is an Akt kinase coactivator. Mol Cell 6:395–407

Liu CG, Calin GA, Meloon B, Gamliel N, Sevignani C, Ferracin M, Dumitru CD, Shimizu M, Zupo S, Dono M, Alder H, Bullrich F, Negrini M, Croce CM (2004) An oligonucleotide microchip for genome-wide microRNA profiling in human and mouse tissues. Proc Natl Acad Sci U S A 101:9740–9744

Liu Y, Corcoran M, Rasool O, Ivanova G, Ibbotson R, Grander D, Iyengar A, Baranova A, Kashuba V, Merup M, Wu X, Gardiner A, Mullenbach R, Poltaraus A, Hultstrom AL, Juliusson G, Chapman R, Tiller M, Cotter F, Gahrton G, Yankovsky N, Zabarovsky E, Einhorn S, Oscier D (1997) Cloning of two candidate tumor suppressor genes within a 10 kb region on chromosome 13q14, frequently deleted in chronic lymphocytic leukemia. Oncogene 15:2463–2473

Liu ZG, Smith SW, McLaughlin KA, Schwartz LM, Osborne BA (1994) Apoptotic signals delivered through the T-cell receptor of a T-cell hybrid require the immediate-early gene nur77. Nature 367:281–284

Mabuchi H, Fujii H, Calin G, Alder H, Negrini M, Rassenti L, Kipps TJ, Bullrich F, Croce CM (2001) Cloning and characterization of CLLD6, CLLD7, and CLLD8, novel candidate genes for leukemogenesis at chromosome 13q14, a region commonly deleted in B-cell chronic lymphocytic leukemia. Cancer Res 61:2870–2877

Madani A, Choukroun V, Soulier J, Cacheux V, Claisse JF, Valensi F, Daliphard S, Cazin B, Levy V, Leblond V, Daniel MT, Sigaux F, Stern MH (1996) Expression of p13MTCP1 is restricted to mature T-cell proliferations with t(X;14) translocations. Blood 87:1923–1927

Masuyama N, Oishi K, Mori Y, Ueno T, Takahama Y, Gotoh Y (2001) Akt inhibits the orphan nuclear receptor Nur77 and T-cell apoptosis. J Biol Chem 276:32799–32805

Mertens D, Wolf S, Schroeter P, Schaffner C, Dohner H, Stilgenbauer S, Lichter P (2002) Down-regulation of candidate tumor suppressor genes within chromosome band 13q14.3 is independent of the DNA methylation pattern in B-cell chronic lymphocytic leukemia. Blood 99:4116–4121

Migliazza A, Bosch F, Komatsu H, Cayanis E, Martinotti S, Toniato E, Guccione E, Qu X, Chien M, Murty VV, Gaidano G, Inghirami G, Zhang P, Fischer S, Kalachikov SM, Russo J, Edelman I, Efstratiadis A, Dalla-Favera R (2001) Nucleotide sequence, transcription map, and mutation analysis of the 13q14 chromosomal region deleted in B-cell chronic lymphocytic leukemia. Blood 97:2098–2104

Mok CL, Gil-Gomez G, Williams O, Coles M, Taga S, Tolaini M, Norton T, Kioussis D, Brady HJ (1999) Bad can act as a key regulator of T cell apoptosis and T cell development. J Exp Med 189:575–586

Narducci MG, Virgilio L, Isobe M, Stoppacciaro A, Elli R, Fiorilli M, Carbonari M, Antonelli A, Chessa L, Croce CM (1995) TCL1 oncogene activation in preleukemic T cells from a case of ataxia-telangiectasia. Blood 86:2358–2364

Narducci MG, Pescarmona E, Lazzeri C, Signoretti S, Lavinia AM, Remotti D, Scala E, Baroni CD, Stoppacciaro A, Croce CM, Russo G (2000) Regulation of TCL1 expression in B- and T-cell lymphomas and reactive lymphoid tissues. Cancer Res 60:2095–2100

Oscier DG, Gardiner AC, Mould SJ, Glide S, Davis ZA, Ibbotson RE, Corcoran MM, Chapman RM, Thomas PW, Copplestone JA, Orchard JA, Hamblin TJ (2002) Multivariate analysis of prognostic factors in CLL: clinical stage, IGVH gene mutational status, and loss or mutation of the p53 gene are independent prognostic factors. Blood 100:1177–1184

Ozes ON, Mayo LD, Gustin JA, Pfeffer SR, Pfeffer LM, Donner DB (1999) NF-kappaB activation by tumour necrosis factor requires the Akt serine-threonine kinase. Nature 401:82–85

Paulsen RF, Granas K, Johnsen H, Rolseth V, Sterri S (1995) Three related brain nuclear receptors, NGFI-B, Nurr1, and NOR-1, as transcriptional activators. J Mol Neurosci 6:249–255

Pekarsky Y, Hallas C, Isobe M, Russo G, Croce CM (1999) Abnormalities at 14q32.1 in T cell malignancies involve two oncogenes. Proc Natl Acad Sci U S A 96:2949–2951

Pekarsky Y, Koval A, Hallas C, Bichi R, Tresini M, Malstrom S, Russo G, Tsichlis P, Croce CM (2000) Tcl1 enhances Akt kinase activity and mediates its nuclear translocation. Proc Natl Acad Sci U S A 97:3028–3033

Pekarsky Y, Hallas C, Palamarchuk A, Koval A, Bullrich F, Hirata Y, Bichi R, Letofsky J, Croce CM (2001) Akt phosphorylates and regulates the orphan nuclear receptor Nur77. Proc Natl Acad Sci U S A 98:3690–3694

Planelles L, Carvalho-Pinto CE, Hardenberg G, Smaniotto S, Savino W, Gomez-Caro R, Alvarez-Mon M, de Jong J, Eldering E, Martinez-A C, Medema JP, Hahne M (2004) APRIL promotes B-1 cell-associated neoplasm. Cancer Cell 6:399–408

Rondeau G, Moreau I, Bezieau S, Petit JL, Heilig R, Fernandez S, Pennarun E, Myers JS, Batzer MA, Moisan JP, Devilder MC (2001) Comprehensive analysis of a large genomic sequence at the putative B-cell chronic lymphocytic leukaemia (B-CLL) tumour suppresser gene locus. Mutat Res 458:55–70

Russo G, Isobe M, Gatti R, Finan J, Batuman O, Huebner K, Nowell PC, Croce CM (1989) Molecular analysis of a t(14;14) translocation in leukemic T-cells of an ataxia telangiectasia patient. Proc Natl Acad Sci U S A 86:602–606

Said JW, Hoyer KK, French SW, Rosenfelt L, Garcia-Lloret M, Koh PJ, Cheng TC, Sulur GG, Pinkus GS, Kuehl WM, Rawlings DJ, Wall R, Teitell MA (2001) TCL1 oncogene expression in B cell subsets from lymphoid hyperplasia and distinct classes of B cell lymphoma. Lab Invest 81:555–564

Sgambati M, Linet M, Devesa S (2001) Chronic lymphocytic leukemia, epidemiological, familial, and genetic aspects. In: Cheson B (ed) Chronic lymphocytic leukemias, 2nd edn, revised and expanded. Marcel Dekker, New York, pp 33–62

Sossey-Alaoui K, Kitamura E, Head K, Cowell JK (2002) Characterization of FAM10A4, a member of the ST13 tumor suppressor gene family that maps to the 13q14.3 region associated with B-Cell leukemia, multiple myeloma, and prostate cancer. Genomics 80:5–7

Stern MH, Soulier J, Rosenzwajg M, Nakahara K, Canki-Klain N, Aurias A, Sigaux F, Kirsch IR (1993) MTCP-1: a novel gene on the human chromosome Xq28 translocated to the T cell receptor alpha/delta locus in mature T cell proliferations. Oncogene 8:2475–2483

Storz G (2002) An expanding universe of noncoding RNAs. Science 296:1260–1263

Teitell M, Damore MA, Sulur GG, Turner DE, Stern MH, Said JW, Denny CT, Wall R (1999) TCL1 oncogene expression in AIDS-related lymphomas and lymphoid tissues. Proc Natl Acad Sci U S A 96:9809–9814

Thick J, Metcalfe JA, Mak YF, Beatty D, Minegishi M, Dyer MJ, Lucas G, Taylor AM (1996) Expression of either the TCL1 oncogene, or transcripts from its homologue MTCP1/c6.1B, in leukaemic and non-leukaemic T cells from ataxia telangiectasia patients. Oncogene 12:379–386

Virgilio L, Isobe M, Narducci MG, Carotenuto P, Camerini B, Kurosawa N, Abbas-ar-Rushdi, Croce CM, Russo G (1993) Chromosome walking on the TCL1 locus involved in T-cell neoplasia. Proc Natl Acad Sci U S A 90:9275–9279

Virgilio L, Narducci MG, Isobe M, Billips LG, Cooper MD, Croce CM, Russo G (1994) Identification of the TCL1 gene involved in T-cell malignancies. Proc Natl Acad Sci U S A 91:12530–12534

Wolf S, Mertens D, Schaffner C, Korz C, Dohner H, Stilgenbauer S, Lichter P (2001) B-cell neoplasia associated gene with multiple splicing (BCMS): the candidate B-CLL gene on 13q14 comprises more than 560 kb covering all critical regions. Hum Mol Genet 10:1275–1285

CTMI (2005) 294:71–89

What Do Somatic Hypermutation and Class Switch Recombination Teach Us About Chronic Lymphocytic Leukaemia Pathogenesis?

P. Oppezzo · G. Dighiero (✉)

Service d'Immuno-Hematologie, Institute Pasteur, 28 rue du Docteur Roux, 75724 Paris Cedex 15, France
dighiero@pasteur.fr

Abstract B-CLL cells express CD5 and IgM/IgD and thus have a mantle zone-like phenotype of naïve cells, which, in normal conditions express unmutated Ig genes. However, recent studies have shown that 50%–70% of CLL harbour somatic mutations of VH genes, as if they had matured in a lymphoid follicle. Interestingly, the presence or absence of somatic hypermutation (SHM) process is associated with the use of particular VH genes. Particular alleles of the V_H1-69 gene and the V_H4-39 gene are preferentially expressed in an unmutated form, while V_H4-34 or the majority of V_H3 family genes frequently contain somatic mutations. The fact that some genes like *V_H1-69* and *V_H3-07* recombine this VH segment to particular JH segments and the restricted use of CDR3 sequences by CLLs expressing the V_H4-39 gene suggest that the observed differences in BCR structure in B-CLL could result from selection by distinct antigenic epitopes. It is currently unclear whether this putative antigen-driven process could occur prior to leukaemic transformation and/or that the precursors were transformed into leukaemic cells at distinct maturational stages. The mutational profile of Ig genes has been shown to be associated with disease prognosis. These results could favour the idea that CLL could correspond to two different diseases that look alike in morphologic and phenotypic terms. In CLL with mutated Ig genes, the proliferating B cell may have transited through germinal centres, the physiologic site of hypermutation, whereas in CLL with unmutated Ig genes the malignant B cell may derive from a pre-germinal centre naïve B cell. Despite these clinical and molecular differences, recent studies on gene expression profiling of B-CLL cells showed that CLL is characterized by a common gene expression signature that is irrespective of Ig mutational status and differs from other lymphoid cancers and normal lymphoid subpopulations, suggesting that CLL cases share a common mechanism of transformation and/or cell of origin. Activation induced cytidine deaminase (AID) plays a key role in SHM and class switch recombination (CSR). However, the mechanisms accounting for AID action and control of its expression remain unclear. In a recent work we have shown that in contrast to normal circulating B-cells, AID transcripts are expressed constitutively in CLL patients undergoing active CSR, but interestingly this expression occurs predominately in unmutated CLL B-cells. These data favour the view that AID protein may act differentially on CSR and SHM pathways, but the role-played by AID in both processes remains to be elucidated. Recent work indicates that AID is expressed in a small fraction of tumoral cells, which could suggest that this small fraction of cells may correspond to B-CLL cells that would have recently experienced an AID-inducing stimulus occurring in a specific microenvironment.

1 Introduction

B-cell chronic lymphocytic leukaemia (B-CLL) is characterized by progressive accumulation of monoclonal B lymphocytes expressing CD5 and CD23 molecules and characteristic low amounts of surface membrane immunoglobulin (Ig) and CD79b molecules [1]. Low expression of B cell receptor (BCR) is the hallmark of the B-CLL lymphocyte [2]. Despite normal transcription and intracellular synthesis of the BCR components, this low expression is accounted for by a defective assembly of the BCR chains, resulting in the presence of unprocessed μ chains and retention of BCR at the intra-cytoplasmic compartment [3, 5]. The accumulation of mature B cells that have escaped programmed cell death and have undergone cell cycle arrest in the G0/G1 phase is characteristic of B-CLL. In contrast with in vivo results, apoptosis occurs after in vitro culture, suggesting a role of the microenvironment on the B-CLL cell survival [6, 7]. However, the data that have accumulated in recent years contributed to refute two long-standing concepts about B-CLL; i.e. that B-CLL is a proliferation of immature, possibly immuno-incompetent lymphocytes and that accumulation of the malignant cells is related to defects in apoptosis rather than to active cell proliferation. The new emerging picture indicates that B-CLL expansion is a dynamic process in which cell proliferation compensates for the cell loss caused by apoptosis. The balance between cell proliferation and cell loss varies in the different subsets of the disease, which have been defined based upon the cell genotypic and phenotypic features, and dictates at least in part the clinical outcome [8]. Elevated levels of the cyclin negative regulator $p27^{Kip1}$ protein [9] could play a role in the accumulation of B cells in early phases of the cell cycle. Unlike other chronic lymphoproliferative disorders,

CLL is characterized by high incidence of hypogammaglobulinaemia [10] and increased incidence of autoimmune disorders directed against blood cells. In contrast to other B cell malignancies, the pathogenesis of CLL remains elusive. The uncertainty about its normal counterpart and the lack of key cytogenetic abnormalities also account for this elusiveness.

During recent years, considerable interest has been devoted to the study of Ig variable (V) region to better delineate critical issues in the history of clonal malignant B cells and in prognosis of the disease. The Igs are heterodimeric proteins composed of two heavy (H) and two light (L) chains. Each H and L chain contains a V domain, which defines the antigen-binding site of the antibody, and a constant domain, which is assumed to play an effector function without changing antigen specificity. Mature B cells, which have completed functional VDJ recombination of both H and L chain genes, express IgM on the surface and migrate to the secondary lymphoid organs such as spleen and lymph nodes where they encounter antigens. B lymphocytes activated by antigen stimulation proliferate vigorously in lymphoid follicles and often form special microenvironments called germinal centres (GCs), where two genetic alterations, namely somatic hypermutation (SHM) and class switch recombination (CSR) take place in the Ig gene loci. SHM takes place in the V region of both H and L chain genes, introducing a million times more point mutations than the genome-wide background. This process followed by selection leads to generation of high-affinity antibodies. CSR replaces the Ig C_H gene to be expressed from $C\mu$ to $C\gamma$, $C\varepsilon$ or $C\alpha$, resulting in switching of antibodies isotype from IgM to IgG, IgE, or IgA, respectively, without changing the antigen specificity. Each isotype determines the manner in which captured antigens are eliminated or the location where the Ig is delivered and accumulated. The analysis of the SHM and CSR processes and the recent discovery of AID (activation induced cytidine deaminase), an enzyme playing a key role in these two events, have offered new tools for better understanding of the malignant B cell history [11].

2 V_H Gene Expression in CLL B Cells

Comparisons of V domains have shown that each V domain contains three regions of extensive sequence variability, termed the complementary determining regions (CDRs), and four regions of relative sequence stability, termed framework regions (FRs). The three L chain CDRs and the three H chain CDRs are juxtaposed to form the antigen-binding site of the antibody, as classically defined. CDRs are preferred targets of SHM when compared to the FRs of the IgV regions, as originally proposed by Wu et al. [12]. Among CDRs there are a few preferred motifs, among which the RGYW motif is approximately twofold more mutated than normal sequences [13, 14]. Thus, the sequence and structure of the antigen-binding site can be altered through SHM leading to a change in the binding affinity and specificity of the antibody [15].

Molecular studies of Ig gene rearrangements in B cell tumours can supply new evidences in the understanding of the process of CLL transformation. An improved knowledge of the site where malignant transformation has occurred and a better comprehension of the role that antigenic stimulation could play in the malignant process are important for understanding the origin of CLL. The vast majority of B-CLL cells expresses CD5 and IgM/IgD and thus has a mantle zone-like phenotype of naïve cells, which in normal conditions express unmutated Ig genes [16]. Initial studies of B-CLL suggested that the V genes of this disease have undergone little, if any, somatic mutation [17]. However, this concept has changed following two studies, an initial publication [18] further confirmed in a larger series [19], that have shown that 50%–70% of CLL harbours somatic mutations of V_H genes, as if they had matured in a lymphoid follicle. Table 1 depicts the results from our group in 145 CLL patients studied for V gene expression according to Binet's staging system. These results demonstrate that the usage of V_H genes is associated with clinical system staging [20]. About 2/3 of stage A patients express mutated genes as compared to only 1/3 among advanced stages of the diseases (stages B and C). Interestingly, the presence or absence of somatic mutations is associated with the use of particular V_H genes (Table 2). In addition to its significant overrepresentation (23 out of 145 cases, 16% as compared to an expected frequency of 2%) $V_H1\text{-}69$ is predominantly expressed in its unmutated form and in advanced forms (stages B and C) of the disease. $V_H4\text{-}39$ was also found to predominate among the unmutated cases (Table 1). In contrast, $V_H3\text{-}23$ was frequently and constantly expressed in its mutated form, and $V_H4\text{-}34$ and $V_H3\text{-}07$ also predominated among mutated cases. These six genes were expressed in 66 out of the 145 patients (46%), which, taking into account that there exist 51 different genes, indicates an important over-expression of these genes. However, when compared to the normal $CD5^+$ repertoire [8], only $V_H1\text{-}69$ and $V_H4\text{-}34$ are statistically over-expressed in B-CLL. The fact that only one allele of the V_H1-69 gene is linked to a long HCDR3 and that $V_H3\text{-}07$ is linked to a short HCDR3 as well as the highly restricted CDR3 segment of CLLs expressing the V_H4-39 gene, suggest that the observed differences in BCR structure in B-CLL could result from selection by distinct antigenic epitopes [21]. In addition, there is a frequent usage of certain V_H/V_L combinations, as demonstrated in a cohort of 5 patients in whom the IgG-expressing B-CLL cells invariably used $V_H4\text{-}39$ in combination with V_K 012-2

Table 1 V_H expression according to Binet staging and mutational profile

Stage A		V_H1	V_H2	V_H3	V_H4	V_H5	V_H6	Total
	Mutated	6	3	34	14	3	3	63
	Unmutated	8	3	9	3	0	1	24
	Total	14	6	43	17	3	4	87
Stages B+C		V_H1	V_H2	V_H3	V_H4	V_H5	V_H6	Total
	Mutated	1	2	11	7	1	0	22
	Unmutated	22	0	7	6	1	0	36
	Total	23	2	18	13	2	0	58

Table 2 Expression of V_H1-69, V_H3-23, V_H4-34, V_H3-7 and V_H4-39 according to mutational profile and Binet clinical staging

	Stage A		Stages B+C		
V_H gene	Mutated	Unmutated	Mutated	Unmutated	Total
V_H1-69	2	2	0	19	23
V_H3-23	8	0	5	0	13
V_H4-34	8	2	1	0	11
V_H3-07	4	0	2	1	7
V_H4-39	1	1	0	5	7
V_H1-02	1	3	0	1	5

gene, both associated with unique HCDR3 and LCDR3 motifs [21]. These gene segments from different patients encode for almost identical IgG antibodies as also documented by molecular modelling studies, suggesting stimulation by a common antigen. A Scandinavian group reported similar data on a cohort of B-CLL that expressed V_H*3-21* (together with a very short HCDR3) invariably in combination with a lambda gene of the V_L3 family [22]. It is currently unclear whether this putative antigen-driven process could occur prior to leukaemic transformation and/or that the precursors were transformed into leukaemic cells at distinct maturational stages [8, 18].

The mutational profile of Ig genes has been shown to be associated with disease prognosis [23–25]. These recent results suggest that there are two types of CLL: one arises from relatively less differentiated (immunologically naïve) B cells with unmutated heavy chain genes, and has a poor prognosis; the other evolves from more differentiated B lymphocytes (memory B cells) with somatically mutated heavy chain genes, and has a good prognosis. The high prognostic significance of the mutational profile of Ig genes raised the

Table 3 Prognosis of CLL patients by associating Binet staging and mutational profile of Ig genes

	% of CLL patients	Median survival	Progression-free survival
Mutated Stage A	40%	Not achieved (75% 12-year survival)	156 months
Unmutated Stage A	19%	97 months	42 months
Mutated Stages B and C	14%	120 months	
Unmutated Stages B and C	27%	78 months	

question as to whether classical Rai [26] and Binet [27] staging systems were still useful in prognostic stratification of this disease. We have recently checked this question in the 145 patients reported in Table 1. Mutated (MT) patients predominated within stage A (72%), while unmutated (UM) among stages B/C (62%). The median overall survival (OS) was 84 months for UM patients and was not achieved for MT cases (70% 12-year survival, $p<0.0001$). Concerning stage A patients, both median OS and progression-free survival (PFS) were significantly shorter for UM when compared to MT patients (respectively, 97 months vs not achieved, $p=0.0017$; and 42 vs 156 months, $p<0.0001$). V_H mutational profile could also segregate stages B and C patients into two groups with different survival patterns (median OS of 78 vs 120 months for UM and MT cases respectively; $p=0.002$). The significant differences observed between MT stage A and stage B/C patients (the same holds true for UM cases) indicate that Binet's classification and V_H genes are independent prognostic variables, and should be most likely complementary (Table 3). These results could favour the idea that CLL could correspond to two different diseases that look alike in morphologic and phenotypic terms. In CLL with mutated Ig genes, the proliferating B cell may have transited through GCs, the physiologic site of hypermutation, whereas in CLL with unmutated Ig genes the malignant B cell may derive from a pre-GC naïve B cell.

Mutated and unmutated CLL patients clearly differ in terms of prognosis and may also differ with respect to oncogenic mechanisms (11q deletions are almost always associated to an unmutated profile). Despite these clinical and molecular differences, recent studies on gene expression profiling of B-CLL cells showed that CLL is characterized by a common gene expression signature that is irrespective of Ig mutational status and differs from other lymphoid cancers and normal lymphoid subpopulations, suggesting that CLL cases share a common mechanism of transformation and/or cellular origin [28, 29]. These results agree with the CLL monotonous phenotypic signature, i.e. BCR under-expression. However, despite sharing a common signature, CLLs expressing mutated and unmutated Ig genes differentially express more than 100 genes. Among these differentially expressed genes, over-expression of zeta-chain-associated protein (ZAP-70) [30], lipoprotein lipase (LPL), BCL-7a, dystrophin and gravin are observed in the aggressive unmutated cases [28, 29], while stable mutated cases over-express NRIP1, a nuclear receptor gene, and the ADAM 29 gene [32]. In addition, a non-supervised hierarchical clustering analysis is able to separate the stable mutated group from the aggressive unmutated one [32]. These results suggest that indolent mutated and aggressive unmutated CLLs constitute two variants of the same disease. The striking differences in clinical outcomes of these two variants remain unexplained. Whether they correspond to differentiation stages at the moment of malignant transformation or whether unmutated forms of the disease are in a more activated form, which favours the proliferative potential of the malignant clone, still elude us. Better signalling when stimulated through the BCR pathway in the latter case [33] and a positive role of CD38 [34] in this signalling could also play a role.

3
CSR in CLL B Cells

The other important recombination process occurring in GCs is CSR. There are five major classes of H constant domains in a mammalian genome (μ,δ, γ, ε and α). B cells are endowed with the ability to recombine the same variable domain from one set of constant domains to another without changing the antigen specificity [35]. The immunoglobulin C_H locus consists of an ordered array of C_H genes [36] each flanked at its 5′ region by a switch (S) region composed of tandem repetitive GC-rich sequences of 1–10 kb sequences with many palindromes [37]. CSR takes place between two S regions, resulting in loop-out deletion of intervening DNA segments as circular DNA [38, 39]. Since the Cμ gene is located at the V_H proximal end of the C_H gene cluster, CSR between Sμ and another S region 5′ to a C_H gene brings that particular C_H gene adjacent to the V_H exon. CSR in the S regions is preceded by transcription of the two S regions starting from the I promoter located 5′ to each S region. Since mutations at splicing donor sites of the transcripts reduce CSR [40], splicing of transcripts appears to be important and gives rise to germline transcripts containing the I and C_H exon sequences. The molecular mechanism of CSR can be divided in four steps: (1) selection of target S region, (2) recognition of target sequence or structure, (3) cleavage by a putative recombinase and (4) repair and ligation. The signal to recombine to a particular switch region comes from the cell surface. Cytokines such as interleukin-4 and appropriate co-stimulation through the CD40 ligand pathway induce the production of sterile transcripts from promoters that are upstream of the targeted switch regions and under their regulation. The result of this process is the ability to recombine the same variable domain from one set of constant domains to another.

B lymphocytes undergo affinity maturation through SHM and CSR. During these distinct stages, B cells become the target of abnormal development, resulting in diverse forms of leukaemias [41]. Although, B-CLL cells have been assumed to be freezed in an immature stage of differentiation [42], in vitro studies have suggested that B-CLL cells are not stationary at this stage of differentiation, since appropriate stimulation can give rise to terminal differentiation [42, 43, 44] and to CSR [45, 46]. In favour of this view, studies in vivo also support that a significant proportion of CLL patients are able to display an active CSR. Therefore in a proportion of cases, the CLL patients indicate that more differentiated CLL variants also exist [47, 48].

The most important mechanism for isotype switching is a deletional recombination between DNA-switch regions, though other mechanisms like trans-splicing [49, 50] and duplication of sister chromatids [48, 51] have been reported to explain the production of double isotype expression in the same cell. In CLL patients a subpopulation of B cells expressing clonal isotype switch are able to exhibit the expression in the same cell of different isotypes sharing the same hypervariable domain (Fig. 1A). As mentioned above, duplication of sister chromatids has been demonstrated in some patients and a trans-splicing mechanism has been suggested for others [48]. Interestingly, the V rearrangement genes in these cells remains unmutated, suggesting that B cells without SHM can proceed to isotype switch, traditionally considered to occur in the GC. Thus the occurrence of CSR without SHM indicates that the processes of differentiation and diversification are not linked [47, 52].

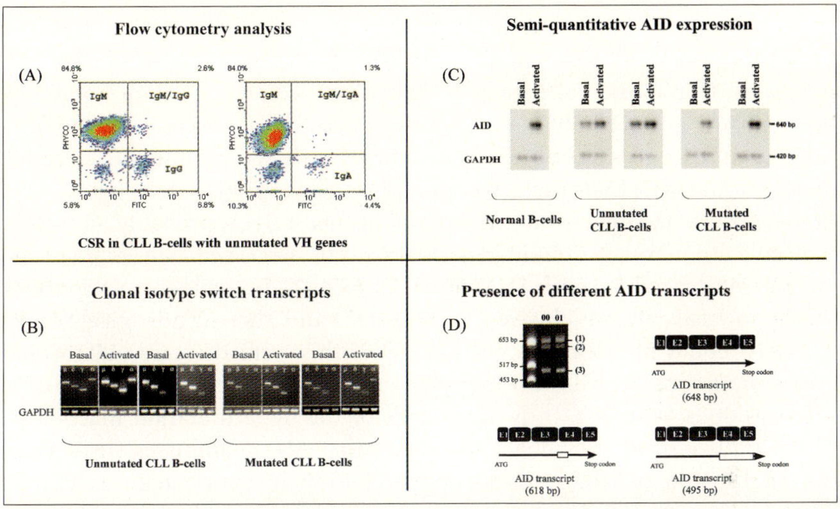

Fig. 1A–D Expression of AID RNA transcripts in CLL and their relation in CSR and SHM process. **A** Flow cytometry analysis: This picture depicts two different CLL patients displaying active CSR. On the *left* a patient displaying a small subset of B cells co-expressing IgM and IgG and a small subset expressing exclusively IgG, On the *right* a patient with IgM and IgA co-expression in a small subset of tumoral cells. **B** Clonal isotype switch transcripts: mRNA transcript amplifications with tumour-related V_H primers in 5′ and Cμ, Cδ, Cγ and Cα in 3′ from unmutated patients and mutated are shown. **C** Semi-quantitative AID expression: The expression of AID transcripts was monitored by semi-quantitative RT-PCR using AID and GAPDH specific primers in the same RT-PCR tube reaction. Representative amplification for normal B cells and either unmutated or mutated CLL B cells are depicted. It is shown that the two patients with unmutated V genes express constitutive AID, whereas in the two mutated patients AID is only expressed upon CD40L stimulation. **D** Presence of different AID RNA transcripts: Normal cDNA and CLL cDNA were amplified and migrated. Three different RNA forms of AID gene were found (*1*, *2*, *3*). The figure depicts a schematic sequence of AID mRNA corresponding to 198 amino acids and the other two variants spliced forms of respectively 618 and 495 bp. Deletions are depicted as *unfilled rectangles*

4
AID Expression in CLL

Under physiological conditions, SHM and CSR occur in a temporal correlation in the GC microenvironment [53, 54]. The recent discovery of AID (activation-induced cytidine deaminase) [55] a protein with expression restricted to developing GCs has revealed an unexpected link between these two processes [11]. Since the absence of AID expression in one form of the hyper-IgM syndrome in humans and in AID gene-targeted mice abolishes both CSR and SHM, this protein is supposed to play a major role in both processes. Honjo and colleagues initially observed an important homology between AID and APOBEC1, the prototype cytidine deaminase, which functions as an RNA-editing enzyme by deaminating deoxycytidine (dC) to create deoxyuridine (dU) [55]. Such evolutionary considerations led the discoverers of the enzyme to suggest that AID might also edit RNA, probably an mRNA molecule ubiquitously present in vertebrate cells, whose editing would create an enzyme crucial for both SHM and CSR (Fig. 2), but evidence supporting this hypothesis remains elusive. On the other hand, there is no logical reason why AID could not deaminate dC to dU. If this were the case, AID would create mutations of dC or the complementary base-paired deoxyguanosine (dG) residues, which is, in fact, the bias of the hypermutation machinery. There are two lines of evidence to suggest that AID deaminates DNA. First, over-expression of AID leads to hypermutation in mammalian as well as bacterial systems [56, 57]. Second, if AID were to create dU in the genome, such residues would eventually need to be removed and the DNA repaired. Uracil–DNA glycosylase (UDG/ung) is one of the main enzymes that remove uracil from the genome, and in its absence SHM is, in fact, affected and CSR is severely impaired [58]. This places AID and UDG/ung in the same pathway, and strongly suggests that UDG/ung removes from the genome the dU created by AID through dC deamination (Fig. 2). Thus, the theory that AID deaminates and edits RNA is being supplanted by the accepted model of an enzyme that targets DNA and, in the process, creates highly mutagenic lesions [59]. In the past 2 years, strong circumstantial evidence has emerged for the role of AID as a DNA mutator. Yet, it is not clear what makes AID predominantly target the transcribed Ig locus. Indiscriminate deamination has the potential to damage the genome: AID over-expression leads to T cell tumours in mice [60], and this expression is a distinctive feature of certain aggressive B cell lymphomas in humans [52]. Obviously, such a mutator would have to be stringently regulated in the cell, and part of this mechanism has been put in evidence recently by Gonda et al. [61]. In this study it has been shown that the balance between Pax5 and Id2 activities has a key role in AID gene expression. At present, some of the most important research endeavours to identify how AID is regulated (what signal cascades are involved), what targets it to the correct loci (particular sequences or certain chromatin modifications) and, finally, what turns the entire reaction off.

Since previous reports [47, 48] demonstrated that an active CSR frequently occurs in CLL, which surprisingly predominates among unmutated B-CLLs, we have examined the link between CSR, SHM and AID expression in CLL B cells. In contrast to normal circulating B lymphocytes, which only express AID

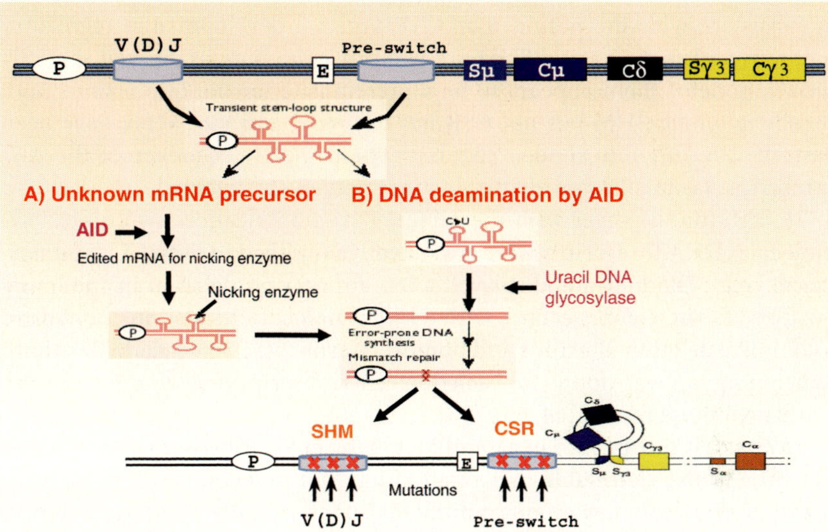

Fig. 2A, B Proposed models for AID molecular function in SHM and CSR: **A** Does AID edit an mRNA precursor for DNA nickase? **B** Does AID directly deaminate cytosine bases?

transcripts following CD40L stimulation, CLL cases were frequently found to constitutively express AID transcripts (Fig. 1B). Interestingly, almost all these cases corresponded to unmutated forms of CLL undergoing an active switch recombination, as attested by identical VDJ sequences associated to different isotypes confirmed by flow cytometry assays (Fig. 1A). In addition, all CLL patients with active CSR and constitutive AID expression are characterized by absence of SHM.

In order to clarify these observations, the pre-switch μ DNA region was sequenced, in search of "somatic-like mutations" usually associated with the expression of AID. Results demonstrated the existence of these mutations, predominating in the 3′ region at a rate of 3×10^{-3}, which was close to previous reports [62] and to the mutational rate observed when normal B cells were stimulated with CD40L+IL-4. In all cases where AID was not expressed before stimulation, it was consistently induced upon this stimulation (Fig. 1B and 1C). However, despite displaying a consistent mutation rate in the pre-switch region following AID stimulation, this did not result in any mutation in the VDJ domain in all CLL cases studied. These results, showing a dissociation between SHM and CSR in CLL, suggest that, at least in this disease, AID would require additional help to carry out the SHM process. Although this evidence is consistent with the notion that AID targets a developmental regulatory pathway, and that CSR and SHM are two processes temporally and spatially linked, none of them appears to be a prerequisite for the other, since both B cells in which SHM but not CSR has occurred and vice versa have been described in different models [52, 63]. The complete sequence of the AID transcript was in all cases identical to that previously reported.

In addition, together with the typical AID amplification, two other low-molecular RNA transcripts were consistently amplified in both CLL and normal B cells. The first one displayed a ten amino acid deletion in the initial portion of exon 4. The second, with a lower molecular transcript, contained a complete deletion of exon 4 and of most of exon 5 (51 amino acid deletion). Splicing signals were found for each different transcript (Fig. 1D). Two studies confirmed these results [64, 65].

In contrast to Oppezzo et al. and McCarthy et al., Albesiano et al. showed that AID is also detectable in a small number of mutated cases, though expression predominates among unmutated ones [65]. By using quantitative polymerase chain reaction (PCR) and limiting dilution studies these authors demonstrated that AID is expressed in a small fraction of the B-CLL clone and that this fraction can vary from patient to patient and from time to time. Since AID can be induced upon CD40L or lipopolysaccharide (LPS) stimulation and follow-up studies also showed that its expression can be down-regulated, the authors propose that this small fraction of cells may correspond to B-CLL cells that would have recently experienced an AID-inducing stimulus occurring in a specific microenvironment. AID is constitutively expressed in a large proportion of follicular lymphomas, diffuse large cell lymphomas and Burkitt lymphomas [66, 67]. In contrast, AID is not constitutively expressed in pre-GC tumours like acute lymphoblastic leukaemia and post-germinal centre B cell tumours like multiple myeloma. In has also been reported to be constitutively expressed in mantle cell lymphoma [68].

5
Concluding Remarks

Although recent studies concluded that CLL constitutes a single disease with a common signature in gene expression, CLL is far from uniform in presentation and clinical course. About one-third of patients never require treatment and have a long survival; in another third an initial indolent phase is followed by progression of the disease; the patients comprising the remaining third have aggressive disease at the outset and need immediate treatment [69]. Significant progress has been recently achieved in the comprehension of disease pathogenesis, yet it raises new enigmas. The elucidation of the mechanisms accounting for the remarkable difference in prognosis of CLLs expressing mutated and unmutated V region genes should be key in the elucidation of the disease pathogenesis.

Comparison of the CLL transcriptional profile with that of normal B lymphocyte subpopulations has revealed that it could resemble resting memory B cells [28, 29]. Although our experimental design [32] was not set up to address the cellular origin of CLL, we attempted to gain insight into the pattern of expression of the discriminating genes between stable-mutated and progressive-unmutated CLLs within normal cells, using data produced by Klein et al. Only a small number of genes clustered clearly to distinct B cell subpopulations. The fact that stable mutated cases over-express genes preferentially transcribed in memory B cells is in agreement with the current B cell neoplasia classification established according to Ig mutational status [70]. Conversely, GC-associated genes were found exclusively within the progressive unmutated group. It is noteworthy that AID, another GC-specific gene, which encodes a protein involved in SHM and CSR, has also been observed to be expressed preferentially in Ig-unmutated CLLs [48, 64]. This suggests that some of the cellular events that occur in GCs such as antigen stimulation, B cell activation and proliferation also occur in progressive unmutated CLLs. However, we found that this group of CLLs also transcribes genes from naïve B cells. Clearly the cellular origin of Ig-unmutated CLL remains to be elucidated. It is plausible that CD38 and ZAP-70 markers, which are associated to this form of CLL, could represent activation markers expressed following the continuous stimulation of the cells by antigens. However, the scenario that has so far emerged is still hypothetical, and it remains elusive whether the state of activation of the cell at the moment of malignant transformation could play an important role in disease evolution. It is an interesting hypothesis that needs to be confirmed.

B cell development can be conveniently divided into an antigen-independent and an antigen-dependent phase. The antigen-independent phase mainly takes place in the bone marrow, where B cell precursors undergo a rearrangement of the different variable gene segments and the initial antibody repertoire is developed. Since these cells have not been exposed to antigen or to T cells in GCs, their heavy and light chain genes display no somatic mutations [48]. Naïve B cells, which are mature B cells, having completed functional VDJ recombination of both H and light L chains leave the bone marrow and enter the peripheral blood as $IgM^{(+)}/IgD^{(+)}$ cells, both isotypes sharing the same hypervariable domain. They migrate to secondary lymphoid organs such as spleen and lymph nodes where they encounter antigens in the presence of antigen-presenting cells and T cells.

Following this stimulation, B lymphocytes proliferate vigorously in lymphoid follicles and often form special microenvironments called GCs, where CSR and SHM have effect in the Ig gene loci.

In CLL B cells with constitutive AID expression, different possibilities can be envisaged to explain the contradiction between the presence of an active CSR and the absence of mutations in Ig VDJ genes: (1) The B cells have arisen from B cells having previously encountered the antigen but remaining unmutated because of an already high affinity for the antigen; (2) the B cells are activated by a T-independent antigen; or (3) the B cells could correspond to true naïve B cells expressing activation antigens like CD27 following malignant transformation. Interestingly, the presence of an $IgM^{(+)}$ $IgD^{(+)}$ $CD27^{(+)}$ B cell subset with somatically mutated Ig receptors has been described among X-linked hyper-IgM patients [71]. These patients are remarkable because they do not express a functional CD40 ligand, cannot switch Ig isotype and do not form GCs and memory B cells. These results could imply that these cells expand and diversify their Ig receptors in the absence of classical cognate T–B collaboration and raise the possibility that a separate diversification pathway could exist [72]. However, it is currently unclear where this putative separate pathway is located and whether it could exist in B-CLL, as postulated by Caligaris Cappio et al. [73], in a pseudofollicular microenvironment where infiltrating autologous T cells can provide CD40 stimulation and cytokines.

Additional studies of mechanisms of SHM and CSR in CLL B cells can provide new clues in the understanding of the process of malignant transformation. They could allow a better definition of the site where malignant transformation has occurred and the putative role that stimulation by the antigen could play in the malignant process.

References

1. Moreau EJ, Matutes E, A'Hern RP, Morilla AM, Morilla RM, Owusu-Ankomah KA, Seon BK, Catovsky D (1997) Improvement of the chronic lymphocytic leukemia scoring system with the monoclonal antibody SN8 (CD79b). Am J Clin Pathol 108:378–382
2. Ternynck T, Dighiero G, Follezou J, Binet JL (1974) Comparison of normal and CLL lymphocyte surface Ig determinants using peroxidase-labeled antibodies. I. Detection and quantitation of light chain determinants. Blood 43:789–795
3. Payelle-Brogard B, Magnac C, Alcover A, Roux P, Dighiero G (2002) Defective assembly of the B-cell receptor chains accounts for its low expression in B-chronic lymphocytic leukaemia. Br J Haematol 118:976–985

4. Payelle-Brogard B, Magnac C, Oppezzo P, Dumas G, Dighiero G, Vuillier F (2003) Retention and defective assembly of the B-cell receptor in the endoplasmic reticulum of chronic lymphocytic leukaemia B cells cannot be reverted upon CD40 ligand stimulation. Leukemia 17:1196–1199
5. Granziero L, Ghia P, Circosta P, Gottardi D, Strola G, Geuna M, Montagna L, Piccoli P, Chilosi M, Caligaris-Cappio F (2001) Survivin is expressed on CD40 stimulation and interfaces proliferation and apoptosis in B-cell chronic lymphocytic leukemia. Blood 97:2777–2783
6. Lagneaux L, Delforge A, De Bruyn C, Bernier M, Bron D (1999) Adhesion to bone marrow stroma inhibits apoptosis of chronic lymphocytic leukemia cells. Leuk Lymphoma 35:445–453
7. Chiorazzi N, Ferrarini M (2003) B cell chronic lymphocytic leukemia: lessons learned from studies of the B cell antigen receptor. Annu Rev Immunol 21:841–894
8. Vrhovac R, Delmer A, Tang R, Marie JP, Zittoun R, Ajchenbaum-Cymbalista F (1998) Prognostic significance of the cell cycle inhibitor p27Kip1 in chronic B-cell lymphocytic leukemia. Blood 91:4694–4700
9. Dighiero G (1988) An attempt to explain disordered immunity and hypogammaglobulinemia in B-CLL. Nouv Rev Fr Hematol 30:283–288
10. Honjo T, Kinoshita K, Muramatsu M (2002) Molecular mechanism of class switch recombination: linkage with somatic hypermutation. Annu Rev Immunol 20:165–196
11. Wu TT, Kabat EA, Bilofsky H (1979) Some sequence similarities among cloned mouse DNA segments that code for lambda and kappa light chains of immunoglobulins. Proc Natl Acad Sci U S A 76:4617–4621
12. Bachl J, Steinberg C, Wabl M (1997) Critical test of hot spot motifs for immunoglobulin hypermutation. Eur J Immunol 27:3398–3403
13. Dorner T, Brezinschek HP, Brezinschek RI, Foster SJ, Domiati-Saad R, Lipsky PE (1997) Analysis of the frequency and pattern of somatic mutations within nonproductively rearranged human variable heavy chain genes. J Immunol 158:2779–2789
14. Jacobs H, Bross L (2001) Towards an understanding of somatic hypermutation. Curr Opin Immunol 13:208–218
15. Pascual V, Liu YJ, Magalski A, de Bouteiller O, Banchereau J, Capra JD (1994) Analysis of somatic mutation in five B cell subsets of human tonsil. J Exp Med 180:329–339
16. Kipps TJ (1993) Immunoglobulin genes in chronic lymphocytic leukemia [see comments]. Blood Cells 19:615–625; discussion 631–612
17. Schroeder HW Jr, Dighiero G (1994) The pathogenesis of chronic lymphocytic leukemia: analysis of the antibody repertoire. Immunol Today 15:288–294
18. Fais F, Ghiotto F, Hashimoto S, Sellars B, Valetto A, Allen SL, Schulman P, Vinciguerra VP, Rai K, Rassenti LZ, et al (1998) Chronic lymphocytic leukemia B cells express restricted sets of mutated and unmutated antigen receptors. J Clin Invest 102:1515–1525
19. Vasconcelos Y, Davi F, Levy V, Oppezzo P, Magnac C, Michel A, Yamamoto M, Pritsch O, Merle-Beral H, Maloum K, et al (2003) Binet's staging system and VH genes are independent but complementary prognostic indicators in chronic lymphocytic leukemia. J Clin Oncol 21:3928–3932

20. Ghiotto F, Fais F, Valetto A, Albesiano E, Hashimoto S, Dono M, Ikematsu H, Allen SL, Kolitz J, Rai KR, et al (2004) Remarkably similar antigen receptors among a subset of patients with chronic lymphocytic leukemia. J Clin Invest 113:1008–1016
21. Tobin G, Thunberg U, Johnson A, Thorn I, Soderberg O, Hultdin M, Botling J, Enblad G, Sallstrom J, Sundstrom C, et al (2002) Somatically mutated Ig V(H)3–21 genes characterize a new subset of chronic lymphocytic leukemia. Blood 99:2262–2264
22. Damle RN, Ghiotto F, Valetto A, Albesiano E, Fais F, Yan XJ, Sison CP, Allen SL, Kolitz J, Schulman P, et al (2002) B-cell chronic lymphocytic leukemia cells express a surface membrane phenotype of activated, antigen-experienced B lymphocytes. Blood 99:4087–4093
23. Hamblin TJ, Davis Z, Gardiner A, Oscier DG, Stevenson FK (1999) Unmutated Ig V(H) genes are associated with a more aggressive form of chronic lymphocytic leukemia. Blood 94:1848–1854
24. Maloum K, Davi F, Merle-Beral H, Pritsch O, Magnac C, Vuillier F, Dighiero G, Troussard X, Mauro FF, Benichou J (2000) Expression of unmutated VH genes is a detrimental prognostic factor in chronic lymphocytic leukemia. Blood 96:377–379
25. Rai KR, Sawitsky A, Cronkite EP, Chanana AD, Levy RN, Pasternack BS (1975) Clinical staging of chronic lymphocytic leukemia. Blood 46:219–234
26. Binet JL, Lepoprier M, Dighiero G, Charron D, D'Athis P, Vaugier G, Beral HM, Natali JC, Raphael M, Nizet B, et al (1977) A clinical staging system for chronic lymphocytic leukemia: prognostic significance. Cancer 40:855–864
27. Klein U, Tu Y, Stolovitzky GA, Mattioli M, Cattoretti G, Husson H, Freedman A, Inghirami G, Cro L, Baldini L, et al (2001) Gene expression profiling of B cell chronic lymphocytic leukemia reveals a homogeneous phenotype related to memory B cells. J Exp Med 194:1625–1638
28. Rosenwald A, Alizadeh AA, Widhopf G, Simon R, Davis RE, Yu X, Yang L, Pickeral OK, Rassenti LZ, Powell J, et al (2001) Relation of gene expression phenotype to immunoglobulin mutation genotype in B cell chronic lymphocytic leukemia. J Exp Med 194:1639–1647
29. Wiestner A, Rosenwald A, Barry TS, Wright G, Davis RE, Henrickson SE, Zhao H, Ibbotson RE, Orchard JA, Davis Z, et al (2003) ZAP-70 expression identifies a chronic lymphocytic leukemia subtype with unmutated immunoglobulin genes, inferior clinical outcome, and distinct gene expression profile. Blood 101:4944–4945
30. Vasconcelos Y, Vos JD, Vallat L, Rème T, Lalanne AI, Wanherdrick K, Michel A, Oppezzo P, Magnac C, Maloum K, et al (2005) Genes involved in B-cell receptor activation, cytoskeleton organisation and microenvironment interactions are expressed differentially in stable Ig-mutated and progressive Ig-unmutated chronic lymphocytic leukemia. Leukemia (in press)
31. Lanham S, Hamblin T, Oscier D, Ibbotson R, Stevenson F, Packham G (2003) Differential signaling via surface IgM is associated with VH gene mutational status and CD38 expression in chronic lymphocytic leukemia. Blood 101:1087–1093
32. Chen L, Widhopf G, Huynh L, Rassenti L, Rai KR, Weiss A, Kipps TJ (2002) Expression of ZAP-70 is associated with increased B-cell receptor signaling in chronic lymphocytic leukemia. Blood 100:4609–4614

33. Pritsch O, Hudry-Clergeon G, Buckle M, Petillot Y, Bouvet JP, Gagnon J, Dighiero G (1996) Can immunoglobulin C(H)1 constant region domain modulate antigen binding affinity of antibodies? J Clin Invest 98:2235–2243
34. Shimizu A, Takahashi N, Yaoita Y, Honjo T (1982) Organization of the constant-region gene family of the mouse immunoglobulin heavy chain. Cell 28:499–506
35. Kinoshita K, Honjo T (2001) Linking class-switch recombination with somatic hypermutation. Nat Rev Mol Cell Biol 2:493–503
36. Iwasato T, Shimizu A, Honjo T, Yamagishi H (1990) Circular DNA is excised by immunoglobulin class switch recombination. Cell 62:143–149
37. Matsuoka M, Yoshida K, Maeda T, Usuda S, Sakano H (1990) Switch circular DNA formed in cytokine-treated mouse splenocytes: evidence for intramolecular DNA deletion in immunoglobulin class switching. Cell 62:135–142
38. Lorenz M, Jung S, Radbruch A (1995) Switch transcripts in immunoglobulin class switching. Science 267:1825–1828
39. Sawyers CL, Denny CT, Witte ON (1991) Leukemia and the disruption of normal hematopoiesis. Cell 64:337–350
40. Dighiero G, Travade P, Chevret S, Fenaux P, Chastang C, Binet JL (1991) B-cell chronic lymphocytic leukemia: present status and future directions. French Cooperative Group on CLL. Blood 78:1901–1914
41. Fu SM, Chiorazzi N, Kunkel HG, Halper JP, Harris SR (1978) Induction of in vitro differentiation and immunoglobulin synthesis of human leukemic B lymphocytes. J Exp Med 148:1570–1578
42. Totterman TH, Nilsson K, Sundstrom C (1980) Phorbol ester-induced differentiation of chronic lymphocytic leukaemia cells. Nature 288:176–178
43. Juliusson G, Robert KH, Hammarstrom L, Smith CI, Biberfeld G, Gahrton G (1983) Mitogen-induced switching of immunoglobulin heavy-chain class secretion in chronic B-lymphocytic leukaemia and immunocytoma cell populations. Scand J Immunol 17:51–59
44. Sarfati M, Luo H, Delespesse G (1989) IgE synthesis by chronic lymphocytic leukemia cells. J Exp Med 170:1775–1780
45. Fais F, Sellars B, Ghiotto F, Yan XJ, Dono M, Allen SL, Budman D, Dittmar K, Kolitz J, Lichtman SM, et al (1996) Examples of in vivo isotype class switching in IgM+ chronic lymphocytic leukemia B cells. J Clin Invest 98:1659–1666
46. Oppezzo P, Magnac C, Bianchi S, Vuillier F, Tiscornia A, Dumas G, Payelle-Brogard B, Ajchenbaum-Cymbalista F, Dighiero G, Pritsch O (2002) Do CLL B-cells correspond to naive or memory B-lymphocytes. Leukemia 16:2438–2446
47. Sideras P, Mizuta TR, Kanamori H, Suzuki N, Okamoto M, Kuze K, Ohno H, Doi S, Fukuhara S, Hassan MS, et al (1989) Production of sterile transcripts of C gamma genes in an IgM-producing human neoplastic B cell line that switches to IgG-producing cells. Int Immunol 1:631–642
48. Fujieda S, Lin YQ, Saxon A, Zhang K (1996) Multiple types of chimeric germ-line Ig heavy chain transcripts in human B cells: evidence for trans-splicing of human Ig RNA. J Immunol 157:3450–3459
49. Mizuta TR, Suzuki N, Shimizu A, Honjo T (1991) Duplicated variable region genes account for double isotype expression in a human leukemic B-cell line that gives rise to single isotype-expressing cells. J Biol Chem 266:12514–12521

50. Oppezzo P, Vuillier F, Vasconcelos Y, Dumas G, Magnac C, Payelle-Brogard B, Pritsch O, Dighiero G (2003) Chronic lymphocytic leukemia B cells expressing AID display a dissociation between class switch recombination and somatic hypermutation. Blood 9:9
51. Gearhart PJ, Johnson ND, Douglas R, Hood L (1981) IgG antibodies to phosphorylcholine exhibit more diversity than their IgM counterparts. Nature 291:29–34
52. Siekevitz M, Kocks C, Rajewsky K, Dildrop R (1987) Analysis of somatic mutation and class switching in naive and memory B cells generating adoptive primary and secondary responses. Cell 48:757–770
53. Muramatsu M, Sankaranand VS, Anant S, Sugai M, Kinoshita K, Davidson NO, Honjo T (1999) Specific expression of activation-induced cytidine deaminase (AID), a novel member of the RNA-editing deaminase family in germinal center B cells. J Biol Chem 274:18470–18476
54. Yoshikawa K, Okazaki IM, Eto T, Kinoshita K, Muramatsu M, Nagaoka H, Honjo T (2002) AID enzyme-induced hypermutation in an actively transcribed gene in fibroblasts. Science 296:2033–2036
55. Petersen-Mahrt SK, Harris RS, Neuberger MS (2002) AID mutates E. coli suggesting a DNA deamination mechanism for antibody diversification. Nature 418:99–103
56. Rada C, Williams GT, Nilsen H, Barnes DE, Lindahl T, Neuberger MS (2002) Immunoglobulin isotype switching is inhibited and somatic hypermutation perturbed in UNG-deficient mice. Curr Biol 12:1748–1755
57. Besmer E, Gourzi P, Papavasiliou FN (2004) The regulation of somatic hypermutation. Curr Opin Immunol 16:241–245
58. Okazaki IM, Hiai H, Kakazu N, Yamada S, Muramatsu M, Kinoshita K, Honjo T (2003) Constitutive expression of AID leads to tumorigenesis. J Exp Med 197:1173–1181
59. Gonda H, Sugai M, Nambu Y, Katakai T, Agata Y, Mori KJ, Yokota Y, Shimizu A (2003) The balance between Pax5 and Id2 activities is the key to AID gene expression. J Exp Med 198:1427–1437
60. Nagaoka H, Muramatsu M, Yamamura N, Kinoshita K, Honjo T (2002) Activation-induced deaminase (AID)-directed hypermutation in the immunoglobulin Smu region: implication of AID involvement in a common step of class switch recombination and somatic hypermutation. J Exp Med 195:529–534
61. Honjo T (2002) Does AID need another aid? Nat Immunol 3:800–801
62. McCarthy H, Wierda WG, Barron LL, Cromwell CC, Wang J, Coombes KR, Rangel R, Elenitoba-Johnson KS, Keating MJ, Abruzzo LV (2003) High expression of activation-induced cytidine deaminase (AID) and splice variants is a distinctive feature of poor-prognosis chronic lymphocytic leukemia. Blood 101:4903–4908
63. Albesiano E, Messmer BT, Damle RN, Allen SL, Rai KR, Chiorazzi N (2003) Activation-induced cytidine deaminase in chronic lymphocytic leukemia B cells: expression as multiple forms in a dynamic, variably sized fraction of the clone. Blood 102:3333–3339
64. Greeve J, Philipsen A, Krause K, Klapper W, Heidorn K, Castle BE, Janda J, Marcu KB, Parwaresch R (2003) Expression of activation-induced cytidine deaminase in human B-cell non-Hodgkin lymphomas. Blood 101:3574–3580

65. Smit LA, Bende RJ, Aten J, Guikema JE, Aarts WM, van Noesel CJ (2003) Expression of activation-induced cytidine deaminase is confined to B-cell non-Hodgkin's lymphomas of germinal-center phenotype. Cancer Res 63:3894–3898
66. Babbage G, Garand R, Robillard N, Zojer N, Stevenson FK, Sahota SS (2004) Mantle cell lymphoma with t(11;14) and unmutated or mutated VH genes expresses AID and undergoes isotype switch events. Blood 103:2795–2798
67. Dighiero G, Maloum K, Desablens B, Cazin B, Navarro M, Leblay R, Leporrier M, Jaubert J, Lepeu G, Dreyfus B, et al (1998) Chlorambucil in indolent chronic lymphocytic leukemia. French Cooperative Group on Chronic Lymphocytic Leukemia. N Engl J Med 338:1506–1514
68. Kuppers R, Fischer U, Rajewsky K, Gause A (1992) Immunoglobulin heavy and light chain gene sequences of a human CD5 positive immunocytoma and sequences of four novel VHIII germline genes. Immunol Lett 34:57–62
69. Weller S, Faili A, Garcia C, Braun MC, Le Deist FF, de Saint Basile GG, Hermine O, Fischer A, Reynaud CA, Weill JC (2001) CD40-CD40L independent Ig gene hypermutation suggests a second B cell diversification pathway in humans. Proc Natl Acad Sci U S A 98:1166–1170
70. Agematsu K, Nagumo H, Shinozaki K, Hokibara S, Yasui K, Terada K, Kawamura N, Toba T, Nonoyama S, Ochs HD, et al (1998) Absence of IgD-CD27(+) memory B cell population in X-linked hyper-IgM syndrome. J Clin Invest 102:853–860
71. Caligaris-Cappio F, Hamblin TJ (1999) B-cell chronic lymphocytic leukemia. A bird of a different feather. J Clin Oncol 17:399–408

CTMI (2005) 294:91–107

Chronic Lymphocytic Leukaemia: A Review of the Immuno-architecture

S. Rosati (✉) · Ph. M. Kluin

Department of Pathology and Laboratory Medicine, Groningen University Medical Centre, Hanzeplein 1, 9700 RB Groningen, The Netherlands
s.rosati@acggn.umcg.nl

Abstract Immunophenotyping of B cell chronic lymphocytic leukaemia (B-CLL) is usually performed by flow cytometry on cell suspensions obtained from peripheral blood, bone marrow or biopsied tissue. Immunohistochemical analysis on routine sections is less commonly performed; however, this approach allows the pathologist and the researcher to appreciate the immuno-architecture of the involved tissues and to gain insight into some of the events that influence the biology of the disease. In this review the authors focus on the following issues: immuno-architecture of the proliferation centres, expression of CD23, MUM1/IRF-4 and cyclin D1, tyrosine phosphorylation and detection of the ZAP-70 kinase. Whenever possible, an attempt is made to interpret the immunohistochemical findings from a functional point of view.

1 Introduction

Immunophenotyping of B cell chronic lymphocytic leukaemia (B-CLL) is most commonly performed by flow cytometry on cell suspensions obtained from peripheral blood or bone marrow or from cells freshly isolated from the involved tissues. The immunophenotype of CLL is well known and typical for this disease. Considering the wide number of intracellular and surface markers that can be investigated by flow cytometry and that cell suspensions from blood or bone marrow are more easily obtained than tissue samples, tissue immunophenotyping is less frequently performed. On the other side, by highlighting the immuno-architecture of the disease, the immunohistochemical evaluation allows one to gain insight into some of the mechanisms involved in the pathogenesis of this disease. This applies to the microscopic architecture both in the bone marrow and affected lymph nodes. In fact, there is ample evidence that the interactions between the B-CLL cells and the microenvironment of the infiltrated tissues play an important role in favouring the proliferation and survival of the tumour cells, thus underscoring the importance of the investigation of the disease in the tissues. Furthermore, immunohistochemistry may sometimes represent a useful tool to verify experimental hypotheses that are generated by in vitro studies. This review highlights some immunohistochemical features of B-CLL that may be important for the pathogenesis of the disease and may represent areas of further investigation.

1.1 The Proliferation Centres

It is currently accepted that in CLL two interrelated neoplastic cell compartments exist: an "upstream" proliferative compartment located in the involved tissues (bone marrow, spleen, lymph nodes) and a "downstream" accumulative component represented by the cells that recirculate in the peripheral blood, the latter being constantly nourished by the former (Caligaris-Cappio 2003). The proliferative component of the disease consists of the "pseudofollicles" or "proliferation centres (PC)", which are the histological hallmarks of the disease. In fact, these structures form the basis of the typical nodular growth pattern observed in the great majority of tissue biopsies taken from patients with CLL. Many of the characteristics of the PCs have been summarized in recent reviews on B-CLL (Caligaris-Cappio 2003; Stevenson and Caligaris-Cappio 2004). In short, the PCs are aggregates of proliferating "prolymphocytes" and "paraimmunoblasts" in which a distinct component of cycling tumour cells exhibiting positivity for the proliferation marker Ki-67/Mib-1 is present. The number of Ki-67-positive cells in the PCs is always higher than in the areas between them, and the Ki-67 stain is thus useful in outlining the PCs when they are poorly visible in routine sections (Fig. 1). In fact, the size and number of PCs vary from patient to patient, a finding that may be of clinical importance. The term "pseudofollicles" refers to the superficial resemblance that these structures bear to normal germinal centres (GCs). However, in addition to obvious histological differences, the B-CLL cells of the PCs differ from normal GC cells in that they constantly express CD5 and bcl-2 and are $CD10^-$ and bcl-6^-. Interestingly, the cells of the PCs share with GC cells the expression of the anti-apoptotic protein survivin, a member of

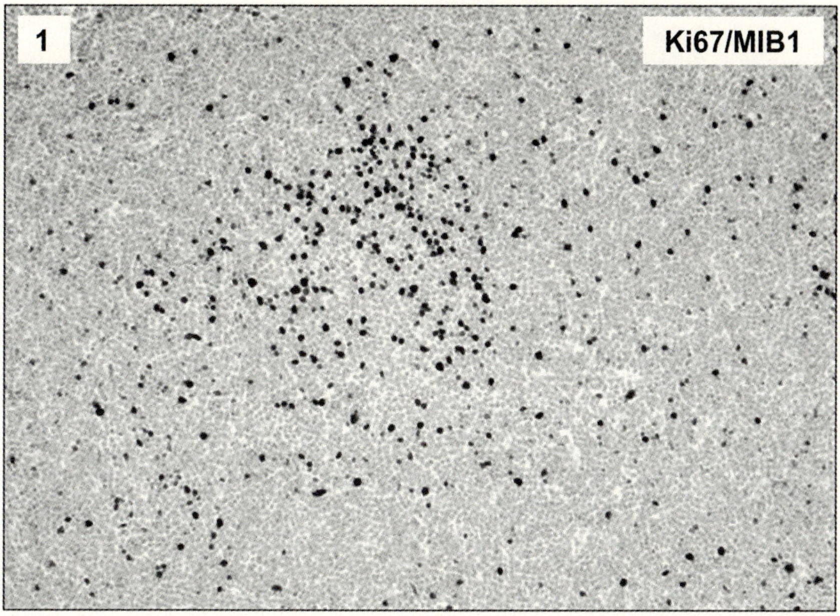

Fig. 1 Ki-67/MIB1 staining of CLL. This low-power microphotograph of an immunohistochemical staining for Ki67/MIB1 (clone MB1, Dako) discloses the accumulation of proliferating cells in the "pseudofollicles" or "proliferation centres" of CLL

the inhibitor of apoptosis (IAP) family, known to have a role in the integration of apoptosis and cell proliferation (Ambrosini et al. 1997; Li et al. 1998; Granziero et al. 2001). Conceivably, expression of survivin contributes to the imbalance between anti- and pro-apoptotic factors that is a well-known feature of B-CLL. Of note, expression of survivin is a feature of the B-CLL cells in the PCs but not in the peripheral blood.

The nature of the PCs and the mechanisms that lead to their formation are poorly understood. It would be tempting to speculate that the PCs are abnormal GC-like structures where the B-CLL cells are subject to antigenic stimulation and subsequent proliferation. The issue, however, is still unclear. Although the presence of follicular dendritic cell (FDC) networks in the PCs has been demonstrated in the early phase of bone marrow involvement (Chilosi et al. 1985), immunostaining of tissues involved by CLL with specific anti-FDC antibodies such as CD21 or CD35 shows a considerable variation in the number and arrangement of FDC networks in individual patients. Several patterns can be seen, ranging from cases showing rather small but still clearly visible FDC networks in the PCs to cases in which the FDC networks are

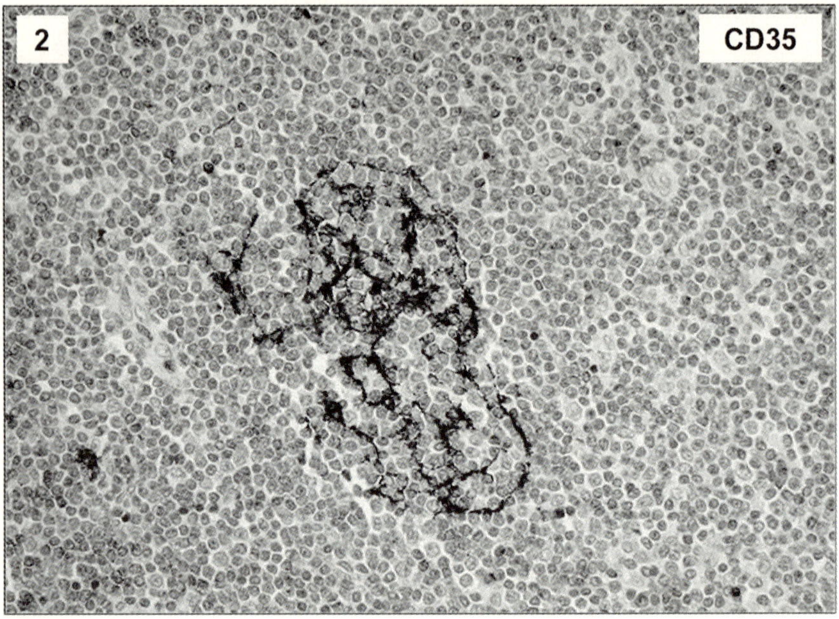

Fig. 2 Follicular dendritic cells in the proliferation centres of CLL: a case of CLL with few proliferation centres that contain small and loose networks of follicular dendritic cells as stained for CD35 (C3bR; clone RLB25 Novocastra). Similar networks could be identified by staining for CD21 (C3dR) but not for CD23. Many CLLs show very few of these networks; however, rare cases contain dense networks and other cases contain residual GCs with these networks next to the presence of proliferation centres without any dendritic cells

fewer, poorly defined and disorganized, or almost completely absent (Fig. 2). Furthermore, in some cases focal FDC networks are seen next to PCs, suggesting that these structures may develop independently. The reasons for this variability are unclear, but it is a fact that PCs can be identified in the tissues involved by CLL even when the FDC networks are scanty or absent.

Experimental data suggest that, in the PCs, complex reciprocal interactions occur between the B-CLL cells and the CLL-associated T cells. By immunohistochemistry it has been shown that most of those T cells are $CD4^+$ T cells that are in close contact with the proliferating Ki-67+B-CLL cells. Some of the T cells in the PCs express CD40L (CD154), i.e. the ligand for the CD40 molecule expressed on the membrane of the B-CLL cells, suggesting that they are activated T cells able to interact with the tumour cells in the PCs. The presence of these T cells in the PCs could be explained by the observation that B-CLL cells from involved tissues—but not from peripheral blood—are able to secrete the T cell-attracting chemokines CCL17 and CCL22 (Ghia et al. 2002). The importance of the in vivo interactions involving the B-CLL cells and the CLL-associated T cells in the PCs is underscored by the fact that several T cell-derived cytokines such as interleukin (IL)-4, interferon (IFN)-alpha and IFN-gamma inhibit B-CLL cell apoptosis by upregulating the expression of the bcl-2 protein (reviewed in Caligaris-Cappio and Hamblin 1999). Furthermore, in vitro stimulation of CD40 protects B-CLL cells from apoptosis (Kitada et al. 1999), induces the expression of survivin (Granziero et al. 2001) and stimulates the mRNA expression of CCL17 and CCL22 and the secretion of CCL22 by the B-CLL cells, which are also able to secrete CCL17 if IL-4 is added to the experimental system (Ghia et al. 2002).

1.2 CD23

Expression of CD23 is one of the immunophenotypic hallmarks of B-CLL. CD23 is a multifunctional molecule that can act as a low-affinity receptor for immunoglobulin (Ig)E, as an adhesion molecule by virtue of its ability to promote T–B cell interactions or homotypic B cell interactions (e.g., via CD21), as a membrane-bound cytokine that can be cleaved to generate soluble fragments with cytokine properties, and as a marker of cellular activation, particularly in B cells (Bonnefoy et al. 1995). CD23 exists in two isoforms: CD23a is restricted to B cells, whereas expression of CD23b is induced by a variety of stimuli (particularly IL-4) on B cells and other haematopoietic cells such as monocytes/macrophages, T cells, eosinophils and platelets (Delespesse et al. 1991). The two isoforms differ in the first nine amino acids of the N-terminal intracytoplasmic region, may have distinct functions (Yokota et al. 1992) and use different signalling pathways: CD23a mediates an increase in intracellular calcium, whereas CD23b upregulates cyclic AMP (cAMP) and inducible nitric oxide synthase (iNOS) (Dugas et al. 1995; Kolb et al. 1994). In normal B cells and in B-CLL, CD23a and CD23b are generated by the alternative use of two distinct promoters in the human *CD23* gene. The pattern of expression of surface CD23 in B cells is determined by a variety of exogenous stimuli that signal via transcription factors that are either able to activate transcription from both promoters or selectively lead to the upregulation of one of the two CD23 isoforms. For instance, the CD23a promoter is responsive to IL-4 [mediated by signal transducer and activator of transcription (STAT)-6], whereas the CD23b promoter is responsive to IL-4, anti-CD40 [mediated by nuclear factor (NF)-kappaB] and anti-mu (Ewart et al. 2002). In addition, the CD23a promoter is specifically activated by the Epstein-Barr virus (EBV) protein EBNA2 (Wang 1991), by the B cell-specific transcription factor Pax-5 (Visan et al. 2003) and by the transcription factor Notch-2. Of note, deregulation of the Notch-2 signalling pathway leading to overexpression of CD23a has been reported in CLL (Hubmann et al. 2002). Nuclear factors of activated T cells (NF-ATs) have been reported to be present in the nuclei of B-CLL cells, and NF-AT-binding sites have been detected in the CD23b promoter (Kneitz et al. 2002). As discussed below, the CD23b promoter may also be activated by IRF-4 and BLIMP-1.

Several groups have addressed the issue of whether in B-CLL the two CD23 isoforms are differentially and/or abnormally regulated by cytokines such as IL-4 and interferons (Fournier et al. 1995; Goller et al. 2002). Although the issue is somehow controversial, the most recent data suggest that CD23 regulation in B-CLL cells differs from normal $CD5^+$ or $CD5^-$ B cells. In B cells, IL-4 is the main inducer of CD23, and its action is repressed by IFN-gamma; in B-CLL IL-4 has a less pronounced effect and the IFN-gamma-mediated CD23 downregulation is lost, suggesting that CD23 expression in B-CLL is deregulated. Regardless of the stimulus or type of B cell used, both isoforms are regulated in parallel, CD23a being the dominant isoform with a ratio CD23a:CD23b of 2–3:1 (Goller et al. 2002). As far as IL-4 is concerned, there is evidence that the B-CLL cell population is "nurtured" by a IL-4-rich microenvironment, whereby the IL-4 secreted by either the CLL-associated T helper cells type 2 or by the B-CLL cells themselves binds to the IL-4 receptor present on the surface of the CLL cells, resulting in phosphorylation of STAT-6 and induction of downstream target genes protecting the cells from apoptosis (reviewed in Kay and Pittner 2003). Other recent results show that in vitro engagement of surface CD23 induces an increase in the expression and activity of iNOS, resulting in an increase in intracellular nitric oxide and protection of the CLL cells from apoptosis (Kolb et al. 2001).

An aspect of the CD23 (de)regulation in B-CLL familiar to the pathologist is the immunohistochemical observation that the CLL cells of the PCs (prolymphocytes and paraimmunoblasts) often stain more intensely than the small B-CLL cells located outside them (Lampert et al. 1991). In fact, in a considerable number of cases staining is only seen in these cells and not in the smaller lymphocytes (Fig. 3); nevertheless, flow cytometry analysis on circulating blood cells is positive in those cases, indicating that this may reflect a matter of methodology and sensitivity of the different assays. Anti-CD23 antibodies reactive in paraffin tissue such as NCL-1B12 (Novocastra, UK) recognize an epitope of CD23 corresponding to the external portion of the CD23 molecule and do not discriminate between the two CD23 isoforms. Yet, from the data mentioned above, it is reasonable to believe that the PCs

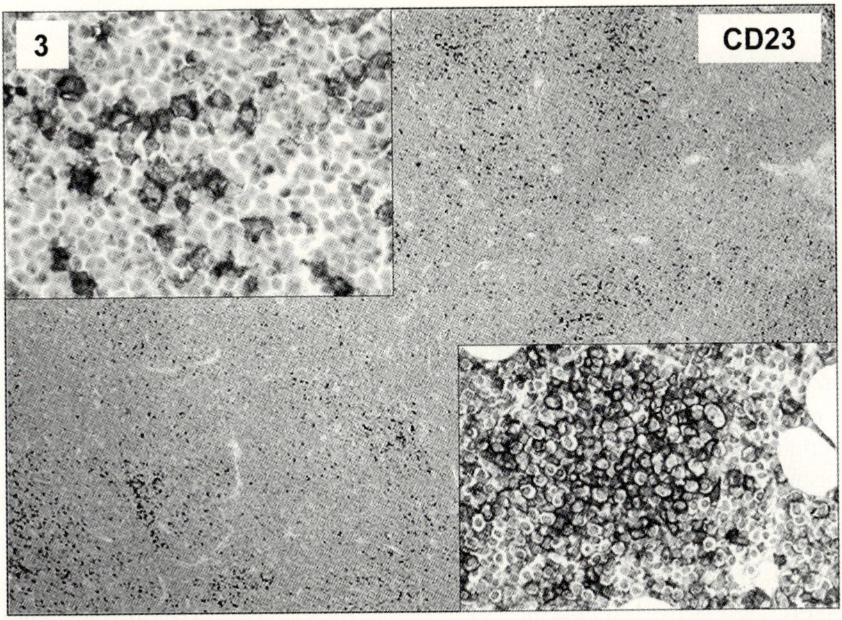

Fig. 3 CD23 in CLL. In many cases of CLL, few CD23-positive cells are seen upon immunohistochemistry (clone 1B12, Novocastra). This low-power microphotograph shows a case with distinct positivity in exclusively a few cells of the proliferation centres. A higher magnification is seen in the *left insert*. Another case shows a very strong staining of almost all neoplastic cells of the proliferation centres (*insert at the right*)

represent the appropriate tissue milieu in which multiple pathogenetic mechanisms (e.g., cytokines, CD40-CD40L interactions) potentially contribute to the upregulation of both CD23 isoforms on the B-CLL cells.

1.3 MUM1/IRF4

MUM1/IRF4 (multiple myeloma 1/interferon regulatory factor 4)/Pip (PU.1 interaction partner) is a recently described protein that is directly involved in B cell development (Eisenbeis et al. 1995, Grossman et al. 1996, Yamagata et al. 1996). Simultaneously, the gene was also found to be involved in chromosomal translocation t(6;14) in multiple myeloma (Iida et al. 1997). IRF4 is a member of larger family of interferon regulatory factors and can be considered as a transcription factor that functions either as a transcriptional activator or repressor (reviewed by Marecki and Fenton 2002). $IRF4^{-/-}$ mice have no detectable B cell response and lack serum Ig, whereas the development of peripheral B cells is blocked on the stage of GCs (Mittrucker et al. 1997, reviewed in Busslinger 2004 and Calame et al. 2003). This B cell defect is multifactorial: In normal precursor B cells, absence of both IRF4 and IRF8 results in the impairment of Ig rearrangement of the light chain genes, a continuous expression of the surrogate light chain B cell receptor and a persistent proliferation of these early precursor B cells (Lu et al. 2003). In mature B cells, IRF4 is highly expressed in a distinct subset of GC B cells that shows transition to plasma cells (Falini et al. 2000). These cells are normally present in the light zone of the GC. In parallel, in vitro studies on mature B cells showed that IRF4 can be induced upon CD40 and IL-4 stimulation (Gupta et al. 1999). IRF4 can exert its function alone or in combination with other partners such as PU.1 , and it can bind to many different enhancer regions, including Ig kappa and lambda enhancers, MHC class I, CIITA (class II transactivator) etc. Association with PU.1 is also essential for activation of CD20. Of interest for CLL, IRF4 is a transactivator of CD23, since it participates in a complex that targets the IFNγ activation site (GAS) (Gupta et al. 2001). This transactivation is blocked by BCL-6. Interestingly, Falini and coworkers found a relatively high expression of IRF4 in approximately half of the CLL cases (Falini et al. 2000) and Ito et al. described a preferential staining of cells within the proliferation centres of CLL (Ito et al. 2002). Since expression of BCl-6 is regularly absent in CLL, these data might suggest that IRF4 drives CD23 expression in the proliferation centres of CLL (Chang et al. 2002 and Ito et al. 2002).

1.4 Cyclin D1

In human lymphoid neoplasms, immunohistochemical detection of cyclin D1 is observed in almost all cases of mantle cell lymphomas and in a subset of multiple myelomas and hairy cell leukemias. The assay is of diagnostic importance since the large majority of mantle cell lymphomas are cyclin D1 positive, whereas, despite sporadic exceptions, other mature small B cell lymphoproliferations, including most cases of B-CLL and splenic marginal zone lymphomas (SMZL), are not. The t(11;14) has been reported in cases of atypical B-CLL (Avet-Loiseau et al. 1998), but some of these cases may actually represent mantle cell lymphomas in leukaemic phase (Matutes et al. 1999). Finally, a considerable part of B cell prolymphocytic leukaemia's carry a t(11;14) with overexpression of cyclin D1, but based on a refined immunophenotypic analysis of these cases, such cases most likely also reflect pure splenomegalic mantle cell lymphomas (Ruchlemer et al. 2004).

Immunohistochemical detection of cyclin D1 using mouse monoclonal an-

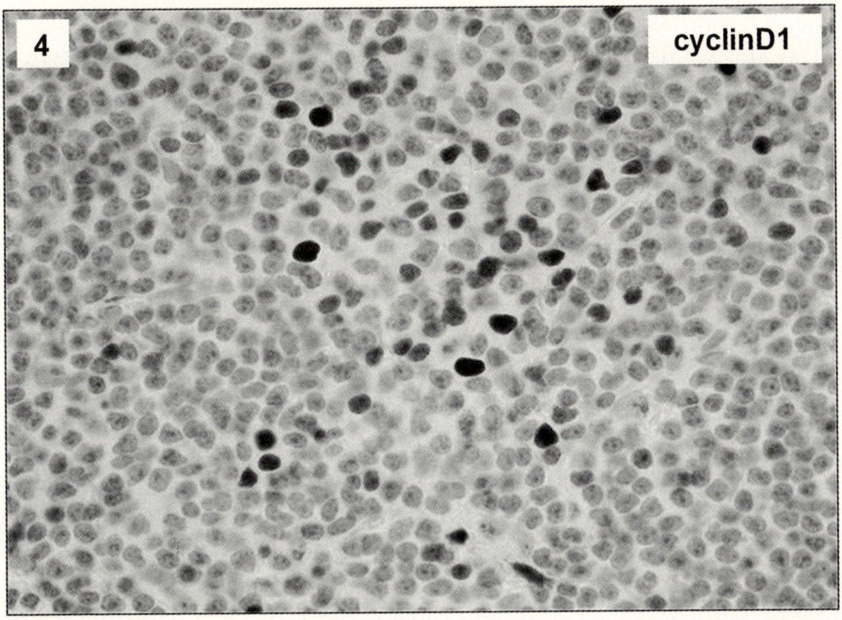

Fig. 4 Cyclin D1 staining in CLL. In very exceptional cases of CLL, the proliferation centres may contain a few cyclin D1 (clone AM29, Zymed) positive cells. The areas in between were completely negative. The two cases tested by us were $CD5^+$ and $CD23^+$ and we could not identify any 11q13/BCL1 breakpoint by fluorescent in situ hybridization (FISH). PCR analysis for IgH rearrangements showed only one peak using framework (FR) I, II and III primers followed by a GeneScan read-out method, making it highly unlikely that the tumour consisted of two clones (one CLL and one mantle cell lymphoma)

tibodies (MAb) can at times be problematic or give equivocal results; however, it is likely that the recent introduction in the immunohistochemical practice of rabbit MAbs raised against cyclin D1 will increase the reliability of the assay. As far as B-CLL is concerned, a recent immunohistochemical study using the rabbit MAb SP4 (LabVision, Fremont, CA) has reported convincing evidence of intranuclear expression of cyclin D1 in a small subset of CLL cases (Cheuk et al. 2004). The authors reported cyclin D1 positivity in 2/15 (13%) B-CLL cases with one of two possible patterns: a diffuse staining in the majority of the tumour cells or positivity in only a proportion of cells in the PCs. In our own experience, B-CLL cases with cyclin D1 positivity are very rare. We have encountered few such cases and observed expression of cyclin D1 only in the prolymphocytes and paraimmunoblasts located in the PCs (Fig. 4). We have not been able to detect the t(11;14) in these cases by means of a highly sensitive fluorescent in situ hybridization (FISH) assay.

At present, there is uncertainty about the mechanisms leading to overexpression of cyclin D1 in these rare cases of CLL and its clinical significance. It is not known whether expression of cyclin D1 in CLL correlates with other important parameters such as mutational status of the IgVH genes. In our hands, the sporadic cyclin D1+CLL cases show immunohistochemical expression of the ZAP-70 protein. However, we have seen too few such cases to draw any certain conclusion.

1.5 Tyrosine Phosphorylation

Tyrosine kinases of both receptor and non-receptor type play a major role in intracellular signal transduction through phosphorylation of tyrosine residues, and dysregulation of the function of tyrosine kinases caused by different mechanisms is implicated in the pathogenesis of human cancer (Blume-Jensen and Hunter 2001; Scheijen and Griffin 2002).

Immunohistochemical staining of routine sections with antibodies raised against phosphorylated tyrosine residues may serve as a useful screening method for the detection of tumours characterized by increased phosphotyrosine levels caused by a dysregulated tyrosine kinase, providing that the normal tissue in which the tumour arises contains only low amounts of phosphotyrosine (Pulford et al. 1999). In normal tonsils and lymph nodes, lymphoid cells are generally weakly stained, whereas endothelial cells and suprabasal squamous epithelial cells are more intensely stained and serve as internal controls (Pulford et al. 1999). This staining pattern suggests that the activity of tyrosine kinases in lymphoid cells is normally subjected to a tight control. There are relatively little data in the literature regarding the reactivity of human lymphomas with anti-phosphotyrosine antibodies. Strong cytoplasmic or, rarely, membranous staining for phosphotyrosine has been reported to be typical of anaplastic large cell lymphomas (ALCL) expressing the anaplastic lymphoma kinase (ALK) (Pulford et al.1999; Haralambieva 2002) known to carry a dysregulated ALK kinase. In the study of Haralambieva et al., lymphoproliferations other than ALK-positive ALCL (including B-CLL) showed a heterogeneous staining pattern, with only a proportion of non-ALCL lymphoid tumours exhibiting variable degrees of membranous staining that were distinctly weaker than in ALK-positive ALCL. In the same study, 4 of 6 cases of B-CLL were reported to exhibit some degree of anti-phosphotyrosine positivity, which was stronger in the pseudofollicles. Such a staining pattern suggests that the moderate increase in phosphotyrosine in B-CLL, and particularly in the cells located in the PCs, could be related to activating stimuli such as cytokines or signalling via the B cell receptor (BCR), rather than being the consequence of a genetic lesion activating a specific oncogenic kinase. Interestingly, Western blot analysis of peripheral blood B-CLL cells with anti-phosphotyrosine antibody has shown that B-CLL cases with unmutated Ig genes show a higher degree of tyrosine phosphorylation following BCR stimulation than CLL cases with mutated Ig genes (Chen et al. 2002; Lanham et al. 2003). It is thus possible that a simple immunohistochemical procedure could help to identify CLL cases characterized by a more aggressive clinical behaviour.

1.6 The ZAP-70 Tyrosine Kinase

Since the original report that overexpression of the *ZAP-70* tyrosine kinase gene in B-CLL is preferentially seen in the cases characterized by absence of somatic mutations of the Ig genes (Rosenwald et al. 2001), and in view of the prognostic relevance of ZAP-70 as assessed by flow cytometry (Wiestner et al. 2003; Crespo et al. 2003; Orchard et al. 2004; Rassenti et al. 2004), it is of interest to focus on the immunohistochemical detection of this kinase in B-CLL and other lymphoproliferations and to investigate the immuno-architecture as well. So far, only a few reports have been published (Crespo et al. 2003; Wiestner et al. 2003; Admirand et al. 2004). Immunohistochemical detection of the ZAP-70 protein in B-CLL may serve as a surrogate for Ig mutational analysis and provide important prognostic information in a quick and cost-effective fashion. Different commercially available antibodies have been utilized. In our laboratory we use the 2F3.2 antibody (Upstate Biotechnology, Charlottesville, VA) with heat-induced antigen retrieval and a Tris-EDTA buffer, pH9. The antibody dilution we use is 1:100. The decalcification procedures affect the detection of ZAP-70, and the dilution may have to be adjusted. Optimal staining requires adequate fixation. Immunoreactivity tends to be weaker or difficult to elicit in paraffin-embedded tissues stored for a long time. In normal lymphoid tissues, ZAP-70 stains intensely the T cells located in the different T cell compartments of the lymph node. Normal T cells show a granular cytoplasmic positivity and sometimes intranuclear staining as well; the nuclear staining may be of different intensity. Notably, the intranuclear localization of the ZAP-70 protein in T cells has been already reported (Sloan-Lancaster et al. 1997). Investigation of the intracellular localization of this protein has showed that ZAP-70 is diffusely located throughout the quiescent cell and accumulates at the plasma membrane following cellular activation, consistent with the notion that ZAP-70 plays an important role in the early events following T cell receptor activation. A considerable amount (about one-third) of the total intracellular ZAP-70 resides constitutively in the nucleus; similarly to cytoplasmic ZAP-70, intranuclear ZAP-70 also becomes phosphorylated after cellular activation, suggesting that it may have kinase activity. The precise role of intranuclear ZAP-70 is unknown; however, its presence in the nucleus suggests that this kinase may have additional as-yet-unknown functions. Interestingly, other protein kinases have been localized to both the cytoplasm and the nucleus, such as c-abl (Sawyers et al. 1994).

Similarly to the criteria that guide the interpretation of the gene microarray data, when evaluating immunohistochemical stains for ZAP-70 in tissue sections of B-CLL cases, it is important to consider the intensity of the stain. In samples from patients with unmutated Ig genes, both the tumour cells and the interspersed reactive T cells (internal controls) show easily detectable reactivity, even though the B-CLL cells often show a weaker reactivity as compared

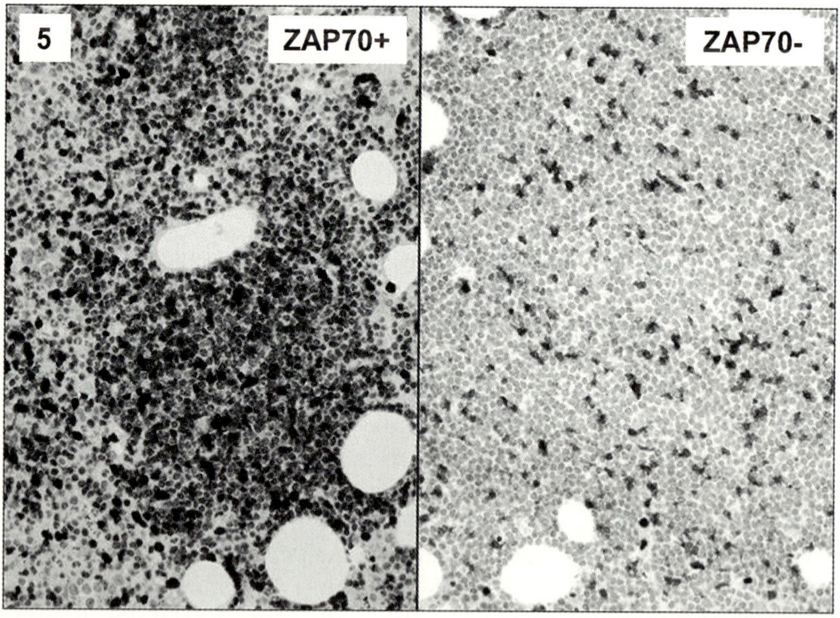

Fig. 5 ZAP-70 staining in CLL. Bone marrow biopsies were fixed overnight in a phosphate buffered saline–10% formalin solution, subsequently decalcified for 24–48 h in a solution of distilled water, 35% formalin and glacial acetic acid (relative proportions: 80:10:10, respectively) and routinely processed. The two biopsies show a respectively ZAP-70 positive (*left*) and negative (*right*) nodular infiltrate of CLL. Immunohistochemistry was performed with the antibody clone 2F3.2 (Upstate). Note that in both cases the T cells stand out against the more weakly positive or negative CLL cells

to the T cells. In samples from patients with mutated Ig genes, the T cells are strongly stained, whereas the tumour cells are either completely negative or very weakly stained (Fig. 5). Based on these criteria, immunohistochemical positivity for ZAP-70 has been reported in about 30%–50% of B-CLL cases altogether, with a strong statistical correlation between overexpression of the protein and absence of somatic mutations of the Ig genes (Wiestner et al. 2003; Admirand et al. 2004): Altogether, 80%–100% of the unmutated cases are ZAP-70 positive by immunohistochemistry, whereas about 10% of the cases with mutated Ig genes may be positive. In other mature B cell neoplasms, ZAP-70 is usually rarely seen; however, reactivity for ZAP-70 has been reported in 13% of mantle cell lymphomas (Admirand 2004), with variable staining intensity. In our own experience, as well as others' (Admirand 2004), mature B cell neoplasms (including CLL) exhibiting ZAP-70 positivity show cytoplasmic staining and at times intranuclear staining as well, paralleling the findings observed in T cells.

As to the function of ZAP-70 in B cells, recent data suggest that ZAP-70 plays an important role in the development of mouse B lymphocyte precursors (Schweighoffer et al. 2003; Meade et al. 2004), a finding that may help to explain the occurrence of immunohistochemical expression of ZAP-70 in the large majority of cases of human acute B cell lymphoblastic leukaemia (Admirand et al. 2004; our own observations). In B-CLL, it has been shown that ZAP-70 can associate with the BCR, suggesting that it may play a role in the enhanced BCR signalling observed in most patients with unmutated Ig genes (Chen et al. 2002).

References

Admirand JH, Rassidakis GZ, Abruzzo LV, Valbuena JR, Jones D, Jeffrey Medeiros L (2004) Immunohistochemical detection of ZAP-70 in 341 cases of non-Hodgkin and Hodgkin lymphoma. Mod Pathol 17:954–961

Ambrosini G, Adida C, Altieri DC (1997) A novel anti-apoptosis gene, survivin, expressed in cancer and lymphoma. Nat Med 3:917–921

Avet-Loiseau H, Garand R, Gaillard F, Daviet A, Mellerin MP, Robillard N, Bouyge I, Arcot S, Batzer M, Talmant P, Harousseau JL, Milpied N, Bataille R (1998) Detection of t(11;14) using interphase molecular cytogenetics in mantle cell lymphoma and atypical chronic lymphocytic leukemia. Genes Chromosomes Cancer 23:175–182

Blume-Jensen P, Hunter T (2001) Oncogenic kinase signalling. Nature 17;411:355–365

Bonnefoy JY, Lecoanet-Henchoz S, Aubry JP, Gauchat JF, Graber P (1995) CD23 and B-cell activation. Curr Opin Immunol 7:355–359

Calame KL, Lin KI, Tunyaplin C (2003) Regulatory mechanisms that determine the development and function of plasma cells. Annu Rev Immunol 21:205–30 [review]

Caligaris-Cappio F (2003) Role of the microenvironment in chronic lymphocytic leukaemia. Br J Haematol 123:380–388
Caligaris-Cappio F, Hamblin TJ (1999) B-cell chronic lymphocytic leukemia: a bird of a different feather. J Clin Oncol 17:399–408
Chang CC, Lorek J, Sabath DE, Li Y, Chitambar CR, Logan B, Kampalath B, Cleveland RP (2002) Expression of MUM1/IRF4 correlates with clinical outcome in patients with B-cell chronic lymphocytic leukemia. Blood 100:4671–4675
Chen L, Widhopf G, Huynh L, Rassenti L, Rai KR, Weiss A, Kipps TJ (2002) Expression of ZAP-70 is associated with increased B-cell receptor signaling in chronic lymphocytic leukemia. Blood 100:4609–4614
Cheuk W, Wong KO, Wong CS, Chan JK (2004) Consistent immunostaining for cyclin D1 can be achieved on a routine basis using a newly available rabbit monoclonal antibody. Am J Surg Pathol 28:801–807
Chilosi M, Pizzolo G, Caligaris-Cappio F, Ambrosetti A, Vinante F, Morittu L, Bonetti F, Fiore-Donati L, Janossy G (1985) Immunohistochemical demonstration of follicular dendritic cells in bone marrow involvement of B-cell chronic lymphocytic leukemia. Cancer 56:328–332
Crespo M, Bosch F, Villamor N, Bellosillo B, Colomer D, Rozman M, Marce S, Lopez-Guillermo A, Campo E, Montserrat E (2003) ZAP-70 expression as a surrogate for immunoglobulin-variable-region mutations in chronic lymphocytic leukemia. N Engl J Med 348:1764–1775
Delespesse G, Suter U, Mossalayi D, Bettler B, Sarfati M, Hofstetter H, Kilcherr E, Debre P, Dalloul A (1991) Expression, structure, and function of the CD23 antigen. Adv Immunol 49:149–191
Dugas B, Mossalayi MD, Damais C, Kolb JP (1995) Nitric oxide production by human monocytes: evidence for a role of CD23. Immunol Today 16:574–580
Eisenbeis CF, Singh H, Storb U (1995) Pip, a novel IRF family member, is a lymphoid-specific, PU.1-dependent transcriptional activator. Genes Dev 9:1377–1387
Ewart MA, Ozanne BW, Cushley W (2002) The CD23a and CD23b proximal promoters display different sensitivities to exogenous stimuli in B lymphocytes. Genes Immun 3:158–164
Falini B, Fizzotti M, Pucciarini A, Bigerna B, Marafioti T, Gambacorta M, Pacini R, Alunni C, Natali-Tanci L, Ugolini B, Sebastiani C, Cattoretti G, Pileri S, Dalla-Favera R, Stein H (2000) A monoclonal antibody (MUM1p) detects expression of the MUM1/IRF4 protein in a subset of germinal center B cells, plasma cells, and activated T cells. Blood 95:2084–2092
Fournier S, Yang LP, Delespesse G, Rubio M, Biron G, Sarfati M (1995) The two CD23 isoforms display differential regulation in chronic lymphocytic leukaemia. Br J Haematol 89:373–379
Ghia P, Strola G, Granziero L, Geuna M, Guida G, Sallusto F, Ruffing N, Montagna L, Piccoli P, Chilosi M, Caligaris-Cappio F (2002) Chronic lymphocytic leukemia B cells are endowed with the capacity to attract CD4+, CD40L+ T cells by producing CCL22. Eur J Immunol 32:1403–1413
Goller ME, Kneitz C, Mehringer C, Muller K, Jelley-Gibbs DM, Gosselin EJ, Wilhelm M, Tony HP (2002) Regulation of CD23 isoforms on B-chronic lymphocytic leukemia. Leuk Res 26:795–802

Granziero L, Ghia P, Circosta P, Gottardi D, Strola G, Geuna M, Montagna L, Piccoli P, Chilosi M, Caligaris-Cappio F (2001) Survivin is expressed on CD40 stimulation and interfaces proliferation and apoptosis in B-cell chronic lymphocytic leukemia. Blood 97:2777–2783

Grossman A, Mittrucker HW, Nicholl J, Suzuki A, Chung S, Antonio L, Suggs S, Sutherland GR, Siderovski DP, Mak TW (1996) Cloning of human lymphocyte-specific interferon regulatory factor (hLSIRF/hIRF4) and mapping of the gene to 6p23-p25. Genomics 37:229–233

Gupta S, Jiang M, Anthony A, Pernis AB (1999) Lineage-specific modulation of interleukin 4 signaling by interferon regulatory factor 4. J Exp Med 190:1837–1848

Gupta S, Anthony A, Pernis AB (2001) Stage-specific modulation of IFN-regulatory factor 4 function by Kruppel-type zinc finger proteins. J Immunol 166:6104–6111

Haralambieva E, Jones M, Roncador GM, Cerroni L, Lamant L, Ott G, Rosenwald A, Sherman C, Thorner P, Kusec R, Wood KM, Campo E, Falini B, Ramsay A, Marafioti T, Stein H, Kluin PM, Pulford K, Mason DY (2002) Tyrosine phosphorylation in human lymphomas. Histochem J 34:545–552

Hubmann R, Schwarzmeier JD, Shehata M, Hilgarth M, Duechler M, Dettke M, Berger R (2002) Notch2 is involved in the overexpression of CD23 in B-cell chronic lymphocytic leukemia. Blood 99:3742–3747

Iida S, Rao PH, Butler M, Corradini P, Boccadoro M, Klein B, Chaganti RS, Dalla-Favera R (1997) Deregulation of MUM1/IRF4 by chromosomal translocation in multiple myeloma. Nat Genet 17:226–230

Ito M, Iida S, Inagaki H, Tsuboi K, Komatsu H, Yamaguchi M, Nakamura N, Suzuki R, Seto M, Nakamura S, Morishima Y, Ueda R (2002) MUM1/IRF4 expression is an unfavorable prognostic factor in B-cell chronic lymphocytic leukemia (CLL)/small lymphocytic lymphoma (SLL). Jpn J Cancer Res 93:685–694

Kay NE, Pittner BT (2003) IL-4 biology: impact on normal and leukemic CLL B cells. Leuk Lymphoma 44:897–903

Kitada S, Zapata JM, Andreeff M, Reed JC (1999) Bryostatin and CD40-ligand enhance apoptosis resistance and induce expression of cell survival genes in B-cell chronic lymphocytic leukaemia. Br J Haematol 106:995–1004

Kneitz C, Goller M, Tony H, Simon A, Stibbe C, Konig T, Serfling E, Avots A (2002) The CD23b promoter is a target for NF-AT transcription factors in B-CLL cells. Biochim Biophys Acta 1588:41–47

Kolb JP, Abadie A, Proschnicka-Chalufour A, de Gramont A, Poggioli J (1994) CD23-mediated cell signalling. J Lipid Mediat Cell Signal 9:27–35

Kolb JP, Roman V, Mentz F, Zhao H, Rouillard D, Dugas N, Dugas B, Sigaux F (2001) Contribution of nitric oxide to the apoptotic process in human B cell chronic lymphocytic leukaemia. Leuk Lymphoma 40:243–257

Lampert IA, Wotherspoon A, Van Noorden S, Hasserjian RP (1999) High expression of CD23 in the proliferation centers of chronic lymphocytic leukemia in lymph nodes and spleen. Hum Pathol 30:648–654

Lanham S, Hamblin T, Oscier D, Ibbotson R, Stevenson F, Packham G (2003) Differential signaling via surface IgM is associated with VH gene mutational status and CD38 expression in chronic lymphocytic leukaemia. Blood 101:1087–1093

Li F, Ambrosini G, Chu EY, Plescia J, Tognin S, Marchisio PC, Altieri DC (1998) Control of apoptosis and mitotic spindle checkpoint by survivin. Nature 396 :580–584

Marecki S, Fenton MJ (2002) The role of IRF-4 in transcriptional regulation. J Interferon Cytokine Res 22:121–33 [review]

Matutes E, Carrara P, Coignet L, Brito-Babapulle V, Villamor N, Wotherspoon A, Catovsky D (1999) FISH analysis for BCL-1 rearrangements and trisomy 12 helps the diagnosis of atypical B cell leukaemias. Leukemia 13:1721–1726

Meade J, Tybulewicz VL, Turner M (2004) The tyrosine kinase Syk is required for light chain isotype exclusion but dispensable for the negative selection of B cells. Eur J Immunol 34:1102–1110

Mittrucker HW, Matsuyama T, Grossman A, Kundig TM, Potter J, Shahinian A, Wakeham A, Patterson B, Ohashi PS, Mak TW (1997) Requirement for the transcription factor LSIRF/IRF4 for mature B and T lymphocyte function. Science 275:540–543

Orchard JA, Ibbotson RE, Davis Z, Wiestner A, Rosenwald A, Thomas PW, Hamblin TJ, Staudt LM, Oscier DG (2004) ZAP-70 expression and prognosis in chronic lymphocytic leukaemia. Lancet 363:105–111

Pernis AB (2002) The role of IRF-4 in B and T cell activation and differentiation. J Interferon Cytokine Res 22:111–120 [review]

Pulford K, Delsol G, Roncador G, Biddolph S, Jones M, Mason DY (1999) Immunohistochemical screening for oncogenic tyrosine kinase activation. J Pathol 187:588–593

Rassenti LZ, Huynh L, Toy TL, Chen L, Keating MJ, Gribben JG, Neuberg DS, Flinn IW, Rai KR, Byrd JC, Kay NE, Greaves A, Weiss A, Kipps TJ (2004) ZAP-70 compared with immunoglobulin heavy-chain gene mutation status as a predictor of disease progression in chronic lymphocytic leukemia. N Engl J Med 351:893–901

Rosenwald A, Alizadeh AA, Widhopf G, Simon R, Davis RE, Yu X, Yang L, Pickeral OK, Rassenti LZ, Powell J, Botstein D, Byrd JC, Grever MR, Cheson BD, Chiorazzi N, Wilson WH, Kipps TJ, Brown PO, Staudt LM (2001) Relation of gene expression phenotype to immunoglobulin mutation genotype in B cell chronic lymphocytic leukemia. J Exp Med 194:1639–1647

Ruchlemer R, Parry-Jones N, Brito-Babapulle V, Attolico I, Wotherspoon AC, Matutes E, Catovsky D (2004) B-prolymphocytic leukaemia with t(11;14) revisited: a splenomegalic form of mantle cell lymphoma evolving with leukaemia. Br J Haematol 125:330–336

Sawyers CL, McLaughlin J, Goga A, Havlik M, Witte O (1994) The nuclear tyrosine kinase c-Abl negatively regulates cell growth. Cell 77:121–131

Scheijen B, Griffin JD (2002) Tyrosine kinase oncogenes in normal hematopoiesis and hematological disease. Oncogene 21:3314–3333

Schweighoffer E, Vanes L, Mathiot A, Nakamura T, Tybulewicz VL (2003) Unexpected requirement for ZAP-70 in pre-B cell development and allelic exclusion. Immunity 18:523–533

Sloan-Lancaster J, Zhang W, Presley J, Williams BL, Abraham RT, Lippincott-Schwartz J, Samelson LE (1997) Regulation of ZAP-70 intracellular localization: visualization with the green fluorescent protein. J Exp Med 186:1713–1724

Stevenson FK, Caligaris-Cappio F (2004) Chronic lymphocytic leukemia: revelations from the B-cell receptor. Blood 103:4389–4395

Visan I, Goller M, Berberich I, Kneitz C, Tony HP (2003) Pax-5 is a key regulator of the B cell-restricted expression of the CD23a isoform. Eur J Immunol 33:1163–1173

Wang F, Kikutani H, Tsang SF, Kishimoto T, Kieff E (1991) Epstein-Barr virus nuclear protein 2 transactivates a cis-acting CD23 DNA element. J Virol 65:4101–4106

Wiestner A, Rosenwald A, Barry TS, Wright G, Davis RE, Henrickson SE, Zhao H, Ibbotson RE, Orchard JA, Davis Z, Stetler-Stevenson M, Raffeld M, Arthur DC, Marti GE, Wilson WH, Hamblin TJ, Oscier DG, Staudt LM (2003) ZAP-70 expression identifies a chronic lymphocytic leukemia subtype with unmutated immunoglobulin genes, inferior clinical outcome, and distinct gene expression profile. Blood 101:4944–4951

Yamagata T, Nishida J, Tanaka S, Sakai R, Mitani K, Yoshida M, Taniguchi T, Yazaki Y, Hirai H (1996) A novel interferon regulatory factor family transcription factor, ICSAT/Pip/LSIRF, that negatively regulates the activity of interferon-regulated genes. Mol Cell Biol 16:1283–1294

CTMI (2005) 294:109–133

Clinical and Laboratory Parameters That Define Clinically Relevant B-CLL Subgroups

N. Chiorazzi[1] (✉) · S. L. Allen[2] · M. Ferrarini[3]

[1]Institute for Medical Research, North Shore–LIJ Health System, 300 Community Drive, Manhasset, NY 11030, USA
chiorazzi@att.net

[2]Departments of Medicine, North Shore University Hospital and NYU School of Medicine, 300 Community Drive, Manhasset, NY 11030, USA

[3]Division of Medical Oncology C, Istituto Nazionale per la Ricerca sul Cancro, Dipartmento di Oncologia Clinica e Sperimentale, Università di Genova, 16132 Genova, Italy

Abstract B cell-type chronic lymphocytic leukemia (B-CLL) is a heterogeneous disease. This is reflected by the very wide-ranging clinical courses that B-CLL patients experience and by the marked variation in laboratory findings between patients. In this chapter, we will review the various clinical and laboratory parameters that divide B-CLL patients into "subgroups," and correlate the parameters that define them. When feasible, we will also link clinical features to the cellular and genetic characteristics recently defined for these leukemic cells. The discussion is limited to parameters that define phenotypes or subgroups that may relate to disease activity and clinical outcome.

1 Clinical Parameters

1.1 Morphology of the Leukemic Cells

B cell-type chronic lymphocytic leukemia (B-CLL) cells can be divided into two broad subtypes based on morphology—typical and atypical. Typical morphology is defined as small mature-appearing lymphocytes with a large nuclear to cytoplasmic ratio, condensed chromatin with rare nucleoli, and few accompanying atypical cells ($\leq$10%). Cases with atypical morphology have greater than 10% atypical cells, defined in various ways, e.g., prolymphocytes, "cleaved," or "large" lymphocytes, lymphoplasmacytoid cells, paraimmunoblasts (Matutes and Polliack 2000; Mauro et al. 2002; Melo et al. 1986). These cells frequently exhibit more nucleoli and less tightly packed chromatin than "typical" B-CLL cells. Patients presenting at diagnosis with clones exhibiting typical morphology tend to have more benign disease (Economopoulos et al. 1982; Vallespi et al. 1991), while those with atypical morphology often experience a worse clinical course and outcome (Oscier et al. 1997a; Vallespi et al. 1991). These morphologic differences do not have the same prognostic implications when applied to patients in more advanced stages of the disease (Mauro et al. 2002). The lymph node architecture of these two broad groups also differs—patients who exhibit the typical variety have a monomorphic histologic appearance associated with small pseudofollicles, whereas patients with atypical cells have greater numbers of prolymphocytes, paraimmunoblasts, or cells with nuclear irregularities and much larger pseudofollicles (Bonato et al. 1998).

The percentage of prolymphocytes appears to be especially important since it correlates with markers of tumor mass (Vallespi et al. 1991 Melo 1986). Certain chromosomal lesions are more common in patients with higher numbers of prolymphocytes within the leukemic clone, in particular trisomy 12 and abnormalities at 6p (Cuneo et al. 2004; Glassman et al. 1998; Kroft et al. 1997; Matutes et al. 1996; Que et al. 1993). Interestingly, an isolated 13q14 abnormality is more frequent among patients with leukemic cells having a typical appearance, consistent with the finding that this chromosomal lesion by itself is not a detrimental marker, but rather one associated with a somewhat better prognosis (Enno et al. 1979).

Patients with clones made up of significant numbers of large or cleaved lymphocytes often display lymphadenopathy (Molica and Alberti 1988; Orfao et al. 1988). In the bone marrow, these cells are more likely to display cytogenetic abnormalities than are small B-CLL cells. The presence of increased numbers of scattered large cells in the marrow may also presage Richter's transformation (Ma et al. 2004). Large atypical cells are more often $FMC7^+$ than typical CLL cells (Huh et al. 1994; Orfao et al. 1988), although the cleaved variety is not (Gonzalez et al. 2002). The eventual appearance in the blood of blast-like cells, cells in S-phase, and cells expressing the cell-cycling marker Ki-67 are all ominous prognostic findings. These findings are much more likely to occur in cases with significant numbers of atypical leukemic cells (Astsaturov et al. 1997; Cordone et al. 1992; Lanza et al. 1992; Orfao et al. 1992).

1.2 Bone Marrow Infiltration Pattern

The histologic patterns of B-CLL cell infiltration and growth in the bone marrow fall into three broad, somewhat overlapping, categories: nodular, interstitial, and diffuse. In general, the presence of a diffuse pattern heralds a poor clinical course (Mauro et al. 1994; Molica et al. 1990; Montserrat et al. 1996; Pileri et al. 2004), although this has been disputed (Geisler et al. 1996). Studies have yet to be reported that make robust correlations of histologic patterns of leukemic infiltration with the newer markers of clinical outcome [e.g., *Ig* V_H gene mutation status and expression of zeta chain associated protein of 70 kDa (ZAP-70) or CD38].

1.3 Gender

B-CLL is somewhat more common in men than women (~1.5:1.0; Mauro et al. 1994). In addition, men predominate among patients developing the disease at a younger age (e.g., <55 years; Mauro et al. 1999). Furthermore, as a group, males often exhibit a more aggressive form of the disease than females (Cartwright et al. 2002; Catovsky et al. 1989). This is consistent with the observations that B-CLL clones of men fall into the unmutated immunoglobulin (Ig) V_H category more often (Damle et al. 1999; Oscier et al. 2002), and express genes more characteristic of unmutated leukemic cells (Haslinger et al. 2004). Since women who develop B-CLL have an increased frequency of homozygosity for HLA class II loci (Mueller and Machulla 2002), a recessive, gender-specific susceptibility factor for the disease may reside within or near the human MHC class II region.

1.4 Familial Versus Sporadic B-CLL

The occurrence of B-CLL among first-degree family members is higher than expected by chance (Capalbo et al. 2000). In addition, there appears to be a familial aggregation of other chronic lymphoproliferative diseases among relatives of B-CLL patients (Goldin et al. 2004). Although in general there are not major differences between patients with and without a familial history of B-CLL, certain features do characterize familial disease, such as the phenomenon of "anticipation" (Horwitz et al. 1996; Yuille et al. 1998) where the mean age at diagnosis of a familial case is often at least one decade younger than of its forbearer (Ishibe et al. 2001; Wiernik et al. 2001). In addition, there appears to be a greater tendency for the development of second primary tumors among familial CLL cases (Ishibe 2001).

Although genetic studies have yet to identify specific characteristic and causative genes or regions in familial cases, certain tendencies have been found (Goldin 2003). For example, there is an overrepresentation of DRB1 11 alleles in these families (Bevan et al. 2000; Theodorou et al. 2002). In addition, gains and losses in two regions of the X chromosome—Xp11.2-p21 and Xq21-qter—are more common in familial CLL than in sporadic CLL based on comparative genomic hybridization analyses (Summersgill et al. 2002). However, ataxia telangiectasia mutated (*ATM*) gene mutations are not characteristic of familial clustering of the disease (Bevan et al. 1999; Yuille et al. 2002). Finally, studies of the Ig variable region (V) genes expressed by parents and children with B-CLL are confusing since there is no consensus as to the extent to which familial cases share specific V_H gene use (Ishibe et al. 2002; Pritsch et al. 1999; Sakai et al. 2000).

1.5 Lymphocyte Doubling Time

Patients whose absolute lymphocyte counts double in less than 1 year often have a worse clinical course than those whose clone accumulates less quickly (Molica et al. 1990; Montserrat et al. 1986), even in patients in the early clinical stages (Vinolas et al. 1987). Surprisingly, rapid lymphocyte doubling times are seen more frequently in early-stage patients (Binet stage A) than in patients at later stages of the disease (Molica and Alberti 1987).

1.6 In Vivo Measurements of Leukemia Cell Turnover

Since B-CLL can have a slow clinical progression with peripheral blood absolute lymphocyte counts that can remain relatively stable for long periods, the disease has been ascribed primarily to a defect in cell death. However, using a non-radioactive, stable isotopic labeling method that involves the ingestion of deuterated "heavy" water to measure B-CLL cell kinetics in vivo, it has been demonstrated that cell proliferation is an important feature of the disease (Messmer et al. 2005). This observation highlights that B-CLL is not a static disease, resulting simply from accumulation of long-lived lymphocytes, but rather it is a dynamic process, comprising cells that proliferate and die, often at appreciable levels. The birth rates of leukemic cells of patients studied vary between 0.1% to greater than 1.0% of the entire clone per day (Messmer et al. 2005). If one estimates the total clonal burden of a typical B-CLL patient at $\sim 10^{12}$ cells, such birth rates indicate that $\sim 10^{9}$–10^{10} new leukemic cells are produced daily.

Based on these kinetic measurements, patients can be divided into at least two subgroups based on leukemic cell birth rates. Although the numbers of patients studied was modest, those patients having brisker birth rates were much more likely to exhibit active disease or develop progressive disease than those with slower birth rates (Messmer et al. 2005). Correlation of leukemic cell birth rates with other prognostic markers is needed and will require further evaluation of larger patient cohorts.

2 Laboratory Parameters

2.1 Surface Membrane Immunophenotypes

The surface membrane phenotype of B-CLL cells has been studied extensively. These studies have identified certain unifying characteristics exhibited by all clones and a few markers or marker combinations that are expressed by clones from individual patients. The latter variability in expression can be used as subgroup discriminators.

2.1.1 Activation and Memory Markers

B-CLL cells have a surface antigen phenotype that resembles activated, antigen-experienced and/or memory B cells (Baldini et al. 1990; Damle et al. 2002; Marti et al. 1989; Sarfati 1993; Trentin et al. 1997), i.e., over-expression of certain activation markers (e.g., CD23, CD25, CD69, and CD71) and under-expression of molecules characteristically down-regulated after cell triggering and activation (e.g., CD22, CD79b, and IgD), as compared with normal B cells. Furthermore, B-CLL cells uniformly express CD27, an identifier of memory B cells (Cerutti et al. 1996; Damle et al. 2002; Ranheim et al. 1995; van Oers et al. 1993).

However, certain differences exist within this commonality of marker expression, primarily related to the number of cells expressing certain markers subdividing B-CLL cases into distinct phenotypes. These phenotypes correlate, to varying degrees, with Ig V gene mutation subgroups (Damle et al. 2002). For instance, leukemic clones of B-CLL cases without significant numbers of Ig V gene mutations typically have more members expressing CD38, CD69, and CD40. Furthermore, the density of HLA-class II molecules (i.e., HLA-DR) expressed on the cell surfaces of these cells is much higher. In contrast, mutated cases have more cells expressing CD71, CD62L, and CD39. Of note, based on the reciprocal relationship of CD69 and CD71 expression, unmutated B-CLL cells resemble more recently activated B cells than do mutated B-CLL cells (Damle et al. 2002).

The expression of CD38 and an extended phenotype that includes large numbers of CD69- and CD40-expressing cells and a higher density of HLA-DR on these cells denotes a subgroup of patients that experiences a worse clinical course than the subgroup without CD38 expression and with the extended phenotype that includes CD62L, CD71, and CD39 (Damle et al. 2002; Damle et al. 1999). These subgroups also overlap, albeit not exactly, with cases segregated by Ig V_H gene mutation status (Damle et al. 1999). This correlation may be strengthened if different percentages of positive cells are used as the discriminating cutoff (Ghia et al. 2003; Krober et al. 2002) and if different flow cytometric patterns are considered (Ghia et al. 2003). Patients whose leukemic clone exhibits significant numbers of CD38-expressing B cells experience a more aggressive clinical course and shorter survival than those patients with low or absent numbers of $CD38^+$ cells (Damle et al. 1999; Del Poeta et al. 2001; Ghia et al. 2003; Hamblin et al. 2002; Heintel et al. 2001; Ibrahim et al. 2001; Jelinek et al. 2001; Krober et al. 2002; Mainou-Fowler et al. 2004; Oscier et al. 2002).

2.1.2
Membrane Ig and Its Isotypes

B-CLL cells are classically described as expressing lower levels of surface membrane Ig, the B cell's receptor for antigen (BCR), than normal human B cells (Ternynck et al. 1974). This has been interpreted as indicating that B-CLL cells derive from previously triggered B lymphocytes. During or following transformation some leukemic clones may become anergic, while others may continue to be effectively triggered through the BCR (Chiorazzi and Ferrarini

2003; Stevenson and Caligaris-Cappio 2004). Subgroups of B-CLL cells determined by differences in surface membrane Ig density have been proposed and may be clinically relevant, although data supporting this are not yet available.

The leukemic cells of most B-CLL cases (~90%–95%) co-express IgM and IgD in ratios that vary among patients (Aisenberg et al. 1973). In addition, certain cases express switched Ig isotypes, such as IgG and IgA (Aisenberg et al. 1973; Wakai et al. 1994; Ghiotto et al. 2004; Hashimoto et al. 1995). IgG^+ cases are more common than IgA^+ cases and primarily express IgG1 and IgG3. Thus, the isotype of Ig displayed on the cell surface of B-CLL cells also can serve as a subgroup marker. This may have clinical significance since most non-IgM-expressing B-CLL cells harbor significant numbers of Ig V_H gene mutations (Hashimoto et al. 1995; Ghiotto et al. 2004) and have a favorable clinical outcome (Damle et al. 1999; Ghiotto et al. 2004), with a few notable exceptions (Ghiotto et al. 2004).

2.2 Ig V Gene Mutation Status

Since B-CLL cells express the CD5 protein on their surface membrane, it was presumed that these cells would behave similarly to $CD5^+$ B cells in mice (i.e., the B1a B cell subset) and would not accumulate significant numbers of Ig V gene mutations. Initial studies of relatively small cohorts of B-CLL cases supported this concept (Kipps 1989). However, when larger numbers of cases were analyzed, it was documented that such mutations occur in B-CLL cells (Fais et al. 1998; Schroeder and Dighiero 1994) and that the presence of these mutations denotes subgroups of patients with markedly different clinical courses and outcomes (Damle et al. 1999; Hamblin et al. 1999).

Furthermore, the presence or absence of *Ig* V_H mutations in B-CLL cells correlates with the use of specific V_H genes as well as certain characteristics of the V_HDJ_H and V_LJ_L rearrangements identified in these cells. For example, V_H *1-69* (Kipps et al. 1989; Schroeder and Dighiero 1994; Fais et al. 1998;), and in particular its 51p1 allele (Johnson et al. 1997), is virtually always found in an unmutated state in B-CLL cells, whereas V_H *3-07* and V_H *4-34* often contain somatic DNA mutations (Fais et al. 1998). Furthermore, the HCDR3 segments of V_HDJ_H rearrangements involving V_H *1-69* contain specific D and J_H segments that create extended lengths and acidic charges (Fais et al. 1998; Johnson et al. 1997), whereas those rearrangements involving V_H *3-07* comprise different D and J_H segments that yield shorter lengths and less acidic charges (Fais et al. 1998).

Most notable is the association of virtually identical sets of V_HDJ_H and V_LJ_L rearrangements among subgroups of B-CLL patients that most often, although not always, involve cases with little or no V_H and V_L mutations (Tobin et al. 2002, 2003, 2004; Ghiotto et al. 2004; Messmer et al. 2004; Widhopf et al. 2004). These stereotyped rearrangements are also biased in the specific V_H involved (e.g., *3-21*, *4-39*, *1-69*, *4-34*, *5-51*, and others).

As mentioned above, the presence or absence of *Ig* V_H mutations and the use of certain specific genes and gene segment combinations is associated with different clinical outcomes. In general, the absence of mutations is a harbinger of aggressive disease and shorter mean survival times (~8 years vs >24 years; Damle et al. 1999; Hamblin et al. 1999). The precise reason for this correlation is not clear, although it must be related to the tendency for the more clinically ominous cytogenetic abnormalities in B-CLL (i.e., deletions at 17p and 11q) to occur in this subgroup (Oscier et al. 1997b; Krober et al. 2002). In addition, since B-CLL is a clonal disease of B lymphocytes with very biased Ig V gene uses and pairings, a role of antigen binding and triggering through the BCR is highly likely (Chiorazzi and Ferrarini 2003; Stevenson and Caligaris-Cappio 2004). The relative contributions that antigen stimulation plays in the conversion of normal B cells to B-CLL cells and in the amplification and diversification of bona fide leukemia cells are a major focus of ongoing study. In particular, the relative contribution of antigen form and availability, preservation of an appropriate antigen-binding site of the BCR, competency of the BCR signaling pathway, and functional consequences of such signaling are essential questions that require more definitive answers.

2.3 Mutations in the *Bcl-6* Gene

Bcl-6 is a transcriptional repressor protein (Neuberger et al. 1998) that plays an important role in the development of germinal centers, the site where normal B lymphocytes most frequently develop *Ig* V_H somatic hypermutations (SHM). Silencing *Bcl-6* in mice prevents the development of germinal centers (Fukuda et al. 1997; Dalla-Favera et al. 1999). In contrast, animals that over-express this gene frequently develop B cell tumors (Baron et al. 2004), indicating a potential involvement of *Bcl-6* in lymphomagenesis.

Bcl-6 is a target of the SHM process in normal B lymphocytes, as with *Ig* V_H (Pasqualucci et al. 1998; Shen et al. 1998). The 5′ non-coding region of this gene is most often affected by these somatic changes. Several groups have identified mutations in *Bcl-6* in B-CLL (Capello et al. 2000; Pasqualucci et al. 2000; Sahota et al. 2000). Similar to the findings for Ig V gene mutations, DNA changes in this gene divide B-CLL cases into three subgroups. In general, mutations in *Bcl-6* are found in B-CLL cells that express *Ig* V_H mutations (subgroup 1, ~35%), although this relationship is not absolute since some

B-CLL cells display mutations in *Ig* V_H, but not in *Bcl-6* (subgroup 2, ~20%). This finding is consistent with Ig V genes being a preferred target of the SHM machinery over *Bcl*-6. Frequently, neither *Bcl-6* nor *Ig* V_H is mutated (subgroup 3, ~45%). A fourth subgroup in which *Bcl-6* is mutated, but *Ig* V_H is not, has also been reported (Sahota et al. 2000).

Recently, mutations in *Bcl-6* and *Ig* V_H were correlated with clinical findings, laboratory data, cytogenetics, and disease progression in a series of Binet stage A patients (Sarsotti et al. 2004). Surprisingly, those patients whose leukemic cells displayed mutations in both *Bcl-6* and *Ig* V_H had shorter treatment-free intervals than those patients whose cells exhibited mutations in only *Ig* V_H. The presence of mutations in both of these genes does not suggest a better clinical course, as mutations in *Ig* V_H do, but rather marks B-CLL patients with the same level of increased clinical risk as patients without *Ig* V_H mutations. This finding is provocative and requires confirmation. Furthermore, the potential relationship of mutations in both *Ig* V_H and *Bcl-6* to other genetic abnormalities needs to be explored, since one patient in this study (Sarsotti et al. 2004) also displayed deletions of 17p13 (p53 locus) and 11q22 (ATM locus), reminiscent of the finding that disruption of the p53 pathway may lead to the development of Bcl-6-expressing B cell lymphomas (Kusam et al. 2004).

2.4
Zeta Chain Associated Protein of 70 kDa Expression

ZAP-70 is a molecule that is integral to the activation of T lymphocytes and natural killer cells via their surface receptors for antigen (Chan et al. 1992). ZAP-70 is a member of the src family of protein tyrosine kinases that includes other signal transducing molecules critical to B lymphocyte activation such as syk and lyn (Niiro and Clark 2002). Gene expression profiles revealed a more abundant expression of ZAP-70 mRNA in unmutated than mutated B-CLL cells (Rosenwald et al. 2001), and this finding was confirmed at the protein level (Chen et al. 2002; Crespo et al. 2003; Orchard et al. 2004; Wiestner et al. 2003). This was surprising at the time since it was thought that ZAP-70 was not produced by normal B lymphocytes and therefore its expression by B-CLL cells was considered ectopic. Recent evidence, however, suggests that normal B cells can express ZAP-70. Nevertheless, expression of ZAP-70 does provide another measure for constructing B-CLL subgroups. Such subgroups also have clinical relevance since the expression of ZAP-70 in significant numbers of B-CLL cells is an adverse prognostic indicator (Chen et al. 2002; Crespo et al. 2003; Wiestner et al. 2003; Orchard et al. 2004; Rassenti et al. 2004). Finally, the presence of ZAP-70 in B-CLL cells may serve as a reliable surrogate for V_H

gene mutation status since expression of ZAP-70 appears to correlate with the absence of significant levels of *Ig* V_H mutation (Chen et al. 2002; Crespo et al. 2003; Wiestner et al. 2003; Orchard et al. 2004; Rassenti et al. 2004).

2.5 Chromosomal Abnormalities

A single abnormality or discrete sets of DNA abnormalities that induce B-CLL have not been identified. Nevertheless, chromosomal abnormalities are detectable in up to 80% of B-CLL cases (Dohner et al. 2000; Oscier et al. 1990). The most frequent abnormalities are deletions at 13q, 17p, 11q, and 6q, as well as amplification and occasionally complete trisomy of chromosome 12 (Dohner et al. 2000; Krober et al. 2002; Stilgenbauer et al. 2001). These cytogenetic aberrations and combinations thereof also delineate prognostic subgroups of patients. Some of these changes have worse implications for survival than others, with deletions at 17p and 11q being the most ominous (32 months and 79 months median survival, respectively). Surprisingly, 12q trisomy, by itself, does not signal a significantly shortened survival (114 months vs 111 months for a normal karyotype), and 13q deletion alone appears to offer a survival advantage over a normal karyotype (133 months vs 111 months, respectively; Dohner et al. 2000). The latter observation suggests that a gene or genes at this site impact negatively on clinical course. The gene affected by the chromosomal alterations at 11q is often, although not always, *ATM* and that at 17p is *p53*. Both *ATM* and *p53* play an important role in cellular responses to DNA damage, cell cycle progression, and cell death.

The patient subgroups defined by these DNA lesions also relate to those defined by Ig V_H gene mutation status (Krober et al. 2002; Lin et al. 2003) and CD38 expression (Dewald et al. 2003; Ottaggio et al. 2003). As might be expected from the outcomes described above, patients with a 13q deletion overlap, to a significant degree, those in the Ig V_H-mutated subgroup and the $CD38^-$ subgroup, whereas patients with 17p and 11q deletions and trisomy 12 predominantly overlap with those patients in the unmutated and the $CD38^+$ subgroups. However, in patients with clones that exhibit mutated Ig V_H genes and either a 17p or 11q deletion, the chromosomal abnormality determines clinical outcome.

2.6 Gene Expression Profiling

In view of the numerous ways mentioned above that B-CLL cases can be subcategorized, one would anticipate that B-CLL cases should be easily distinguishable based on differences in gene expression. This, however, is not the case (Klein et al. 2001; Rosenwald et al. 2001). Even patients whose leukemic cells differ in Ig V_H gene mutation status and exhibit strikingly different clinical outcomes may exhibit gene expression profiles of remarkable similarity. Indeed, when reasonable levels of stringency are applied to comparisons of gene expression data, only a few genes differ significantly in expression between the two V_H gene-defined subgroups (Klein et al. 2001; Rosenwald et al. 2001). This finding is surprising and has been taken as evidence that B-CLL is a single disease (Rosenwald et al. 2001) that is derived from a single cell type (Klein et al. 2001), i.e., a memory/antigen experienced B cell. Alternatively, the cellular heterogeneity imposed by differences in common or as-yet-not-defined chromosomal abnormalities may preclude a precise determination of gene expression differences (Haslinger et al. 2004).

Nevertheless, those few genes that do differ in expression between the unmutated and mutated subgroups serve as genetic markers of B-CLL subgroups. In particular, ZAP-70, activation-induced C-type lectin, lipoprotein lipase, and a few others accurately identify subgroups of patients that differ not only in Ig V gene mutation status, but also in clinical course (Rosenwald et al. 2001).

2.7
Telomere Length and Telomerase Activity

Telomeres, hexameric nucleotide repeats that protect the ends of chromosomes, shorten with each cell division (Hodes 1999). It is therefore not surprising that telomere length, which serves as an indicator of the proliferative history of cells (Harley 1991), defines subgroups of B-CLL cells, especially when one considers that lymphocyte doubling time and in vivo B-CLL birth rates differ between patients. Leukemic cells from the poor outcome group with limited V_H gene mutation have uniformly shorter telomeres than those from the better outcome group with considerable V gene mutations (Hultdin et al. 2003; Damle et al. 2004).

Telomerase is responsible for restoring telomere length after cell cycling (Blackburn et al. 1989). The level of telomerase activity in unmutated cases, which have shorter telomeres, was significantly higher than that of mutated cases (Damle et al. 2004). Thus, telomerase activity also divides B-CLL cases into subgroups. Those patients with shorter telomeres and more telomerase activity may have a poorer clinical outcome (Bechter et al. 1998; Ishibe et al. 2002), although not all studies have confirmed this observation (Ishibe et al. 2002; Damle et al. 2004). Additional studies with larger patient populations are necessary.

2.8 Competency of BCR Signal Transduction

Even after leukemic transformation, the B-CLL cells of some patients retain the capacity to effectively deliver signals to the cell nucleus via the BCR signaling pathway (Hivroz et al. 1986; Karray et al. 1987; Lankester et al. 1995; Michel et al. 1993). Thus, BCR signaling competency is another measure of B-CLL heterogeneity. Although a comparison of signal transducing capability and clinical course has yet to be reported, there is reason to believe that retention of this capacity will be more frequent in patients with worse clinical outcomes. This speculation comes from the relationship, albeit not absolute, that exists between an effective signal transducing capacity, lack of Ig V gene mutations, and the presence of significant numbers of $CD38^+$ cells (Chen et al. 2002; Lanham et al. 2003; Stevenson and Caligaris-Cappio 2004; Zupo et al. 1996). Furthermore, since some of the B-CLL cases that display virtual identity in V_HDJ_H and/or V_LJ_L rearrangements have the worst clinical courses, a role for ongoing stimulation through a competent BCR signaling pathway seems plausible.

3 Correlations and Unifying Themes

B-CLL is not the relatively simple and uncomplicated disease that it was once thought to be. The complexities of this disease combined with the inadequacies of our knowledge of it do not permit correlation of all of the known phenotypic subgroups into a cogent unifying construct. However, a few principles can be derived from this diverse body of information (Table 1). These relate to the development of the disease and its evolution to a more aggressive entity in certain patients.

The first consideration deals with the occurrence of an initial genetic abnormality in a specific B cell that selects out that individual cell, setting the stage for subsequent genetic lesions that lead to B-CLL. The primary DNA mutation is unknown at this juncture. Based on the observed gender frequency differences in B-CLL, this lesion is presumably more likely to occur in men and a selected subset of women. This abnormality could arise in an immature, classical stem cell, or, alternatively, in a mature B cell belonging to a population with a diverse or biased BCR repertoire. Based on the unique characteristics of the BCRs of B-CLL cells, i.e., biased in V gene use and pairing and containing somatic mutations, it seems likely that this postulated precursor cell would come from a mature population of lymphocytes with very biased BCR structures. These types of biases are seen in the murine

Table 1 Prognostic implications of subgroupings based on clinical and laboratory parameters

Parameter		Clinical course and outcome Better	Worse
Cellular morphology	Typical	✓	
	Atypical	✓	
Bone marrow pattern	Nodular	✓	
	Interstitial	✓	
	Diffuse		✓
Gender	Male		✓
	Female	✓	
Familial B-CLL		Not clear, although early age of onset among first degree relatives is common	
Lymphocyte doubling time	<12 months		✓
	>12 months	✓	
In vivo birth rate	Brisker		✓
	Slower	✓	
Immunophenotype	$CD38^+$		✓
	$CD38^-$	✓	
	IgG^+ or IgA^+	✓ (Compared to IgM^+)	
Ig V_H gene mutation status	None or few		✓
	Significant	✓	
Bcl-6 gene mutations	None or few		✓
	Significant	✓	
	Significant in both *Bcl* – 6 and V_H		✓
ZAP-70 expression	None or few		✓
	Significant	✓	
Chromosomal abnormalities	13q del	✓	
	17p del or 11q del		✓
	Trisomy 12	Probably no different from normal karyotype	
Telomere length	Shorter		✓
	Longer	✓	
Telomerase activity	Higher		✓
	Lower	✓	
BCR signal transduction	Intact		✓
	Impaired	✓	

B1 cell and marginal zone compartments (Fagarasan et al. 2000; Martin and Kearney 2002).

The next steps in the development of the leukemia require amplification of this particular clone. Again, based on the BCR similarities seen in B-CLL, especially among the unmutated variety, the most likely facilitators of this clonal expansion are antigen–BCR interactions of adequate affinity. Presumably, the cell incurring an initial inducing lesion is endowed with a growth advantage over other clones stimulated by the same or other antigens and this permits it to outstrip other cells reactive with the same antigen or one of its immunogenic epitopes. The functional enhancement in growth that has been bestowed could take many forms, such as a more efficient response to anti-apoptotic signals, a more rapid cycling time, a more beneficial set of cell surface molecules that favor access and response to trophic signals from the microenvironment, or a higher level of responsiveness to certain sex hormones, to speculate about just a few.

These interactions with antigen probably need to be repetitive. Therefore, the antigen(s) would need to be either always present (e.g., autoantigens or foreign antigens expressed by commensal organisms or persistent viruses) or intermittently introduced in recurrent exposures, as would occur with an intermittent infection or from an environmental antigen in the geographic area in which the person resides.

However, if these repetitive interactions, along with the help of T lymphocytes and accessory cells recruit the pre-leukemic B cell into a classical (Kelsoe 1994) or non-classical (de Vinuesa et al. 2000; Weller et al. 2001) germinal center reaction that activates the SHM machinery, point mutations in the antigen-binding site of the BCR could occur that might either enhance or abort clonal amplification (Chiorazzi and Ferrarini 2003; Stevenson and Caligaris-Cappio 2004). A change in BCR structure preventing binding of the original antigen to the BCR with adequate affinity to cause the necessary degree of surface membrane Ig crosslinking to fire the signaling cascade could lead to clonal "ignorance," which could explain the lack of clinical progression in the V_H gene-mutated subgroup. Alternatively, other changes in BCR structure could make the cells more susceptible to antigenic stimulation, thus facilitating their expansion, as in the unmutated V_H subgroup, or inducing anergy and suppressing clonal expansion of mutated B-CLL cells. This type of model would be especially likely if the original specificity of the B cell selected for leukemic transformation was both auto- and exo-reactive. B cells that express BCRs with these specificities are enriched in B1 and marginal zone B cell subsets.

The ensuing episodes of cell division would make the pre-leukemic cell vulnerable to the acquisition of additional genetic abnormalities that could provide the clone with even greater growth advantages. At some point in time, when the number of these changes is sufficient, the cell would become leukemic. Nevertheless, the leukemic clone probably remains responsive to signals from the microenvironment delivered via various cell surface receptors (Caligaris-Cappio 2003), thereby avoiding apoptosis and promoting continued clonal expansion.

Finally, continued cycling that may be dependent on or independent of antigenic and microenvironmental drive leads to a series of other genetic changes that determine the course of the disease. Since non-Ig V gene mutations presumably occur with varying frequencies and at different, albeit possibly restricted sites, the consequence for the patient could be detrimental (as with mutations at 17p13, 11q22–23, and 6q21), advantageous (as with mutations at 13q14), or relatively inconsequential (as for trisomy 12 alone). Combinations of these lesions, however, are ominous portents for the eventual outcome. The cells that are most likely to acquire or have acquired these additional changes may be those that appear atypical in morphology, with more open chromatin and increased numbers of nucleoli.

Patients with B-CLL can be segregated into clinically relevant subgroups based on several well-characterized and apparently inter-related parameters. We have outlined the currently known data and attempted to correlate them. Further studies will ultimately allow more precise prognostication based on individual patient clinical, laboratory, and cytogenetic data and will improve our understanding of the pathophysiology and the genetic basis of the disease. The advances that have and continue to emerge in B-CLL are proving to be a model demonstration of the power of translational research.

Acknowledgements We thank the present and past members of the Laboratory of Experimental Immunology, Institute for Medical Research, North Shore–LIJ Health System, of North Shore University Hospital and Long Island Jewish Medical Center, and of the Division of Medical Oncology C, Istituto Nazionale per la Ricerca sul Cancro for the work we have discussed in this manuscript.

These studies were supported in part by RO1 grants CA 81554 and CA 87956 from the National Cancer Institute and a M01 General Clinical Research Center Grant (RR018535) from the National Center for Research Resources, the Associazione Italiana Ricerca sul Cancro (AIRC) and MIUR. The Peter J. Sharp Foundation, The Marks Family Foundation, the Jean Walton Fund for Lymphoma and Myeloma Research, the Joseph Eletto Leukemia Research Fund, the Tebil Foundation, and the Horace W. Goldsmith Foundation also provided support for these studies.

References

Aisenberg AC, Bloch KJ, Long JC (1973) Cell-surface immunoglobulins in chronic lymphocytic leukemia and allied disorders. Am J Med 55:184–191

Astsaturov IA, Samoilova RS, Iakhnina EI, Pivnik AV, Vorobiov AI (1997) The relevance of cytological studies and Ki-67 reactivity to the clinical course of chronic lymphocytic leukemia. Leuk Lymphoma 26:337–342

Baldini L, Cro L, Cortelezzi A, Calori R, Nobili L, Maiolo AT, Polli EE (1990) Immunophenotypes in "classical" B-cell chronic lymphocytic leukemia. Correlation with normal cellular counterpart and clinical findings. Cancer 66:1738–1742

Baron BW, Anastasi J, Montag A, Huo D, Baron RM, Karrison T, Thirman MJ, Subudhi SK, Chin RK, Felsher DW, Fu YX, McKeithan TW, Baron JM (2004) The human BCL6 transgene promotes the development of lymphomas in the mouse. Proc Natl Acad Sci U S A 101:14198–14203

Bechter OE, Eisterer W, Pall G, Hilbe W, Kuhr T, Thaler J (1998) Telomere length and telomerase activity predict survival in patients with B cell chronic lymphocytic leukemia. Cancer Res 58:4918–4922

Bevan S, Catovsky D, Marossy A, Matutes E, Popat S, Antonovic P, Bell A, Berrebi A, Gaminara E, Quabeck K, Ribeiro I, Mauro FR, Stark P, Sykes H, van Dongen J, Wimperis J, Wright S, Yuille MR, Houlston RS (1999) Linkage analysis for ATM in familial B cell chronic lymphocytic leukaemia. Leukemia 13:1497–1500

Bevan S, Catovsky D, Matutes E, Antunovic P, Auger MJ, Ben-Bassat I, Bell A, Berrebi A, Gaminara EJ, Junior ME, Mauro FR, Quabeck K, Rassam SM, Reid C, Ribeiro I, Stark P, van Dongen JJ, Wimperis J, Wright S, Marossy A, Yuille MR, Houlston RS (2000) Linkage analysis for major histocompatibility complex-related genetic susceptibility in familial chronic lymphocytic leukemia. Blood 96:3982–3984

Blackburn EH, Greider CW, Henderson E, Lee MS, Shampay J, Shippen-Lentz D (1989) Recognition and elongation of telomeres by telomerase. Genome 31:553–560

Bonato M, Pittaluga S, Tierens A, Criel A, Verhoef G, Wlodarska I, Vanutysel L, Michaux L, Vandekerckhove P, Van den Berghe H, De Wolf-Peeters C (1998) Lymph node histology in typical and atypical chronic lymphocytic leukemia. Am J Surg Pathol 22:49–56

Caligaris-Cappio F (2003) Role of the microenvironment in chronic lymphocytic leukaemia. Br J Haematol 123:380–388

Capalbo S, Trerotoli P, Ciancio A, Battista C, Serio G, Liso V (2000) Increased risk of lymphoproliferative disorders in relatives of patients with B-cell chronic lymphocytic leukemia: relevance of the degree of familial linkage. Eur J Haematol 65:114–117

Capello D, Fais F, Vivenza D, Migliaretti G, Chiorazzi N, Gaidano G, Ferrarini M (2000) Identification of three subgroups of B cell chronic lymphocytic leukemia based upon mutations of BCL-6 and IgV genes. Leukemia 14:811–815

Cartwright RA, Gurney KA, Moorman AV (2002) Sex ratios and the risks of haematological malignancies. Br J Haematol 118:1071–1077

Catovsky D, Fooks J, Richards S (1989) Prognostic factors in chronic lymphocytic leukaemia: the importance of age, sex and response to treatment in survival. A report from the MRC CLL 1 trial. MRC Working Party on Leukaemia in Adults. Br J Haematol 72:141–149

Cerutti A, Trentin L, Zambello R, Sancetta R, Milani A, Tassinari C, Adami F, Agostini C, Semenzato G (1996) The CD5/CD72 receptor system is coexpressed with several functionally relevant counterstructures on human B cells and delivers a critical signaling activity. J Immunol 157:1854–1862

Chan AC, Iwashima M, Turck CW, Weiss A (1992) ZAP-70: a 70 kd protein-tyrosine kinase that associates with the TCR zeta chain. Cell 71:649–662

Chen L, Widhopf G, Huynh L, Rassenti L, Rai KR, Weiss A, Kipps TJ (2002) Expression of ZAP-70 is associated with increased B-cell receptor signaling in chronic lymphocytic leukemia. Blood 100:4609–4614

Chiorazzi N, Ferrarini M (2003) B cell chronic lymphocytic leukemia: lessons learned from studies of the B cell antigen receptor. Annu Rev Immunol 21:841–894

Cordone I, Matutes E, Catovsky D (1992) Monoclonal antibody Ki-67 identifies B and T cells in cycle in chronic lymphocytic leukemia: correlation with disease activity. Leukemia 6:902–906

Crespo M, Bosch F, Villamor N, Bellosillo B, Colomer D, Rozman M, Marce S, Lopez-Guillermo A, Campo E, Montserrat E (2003) ZAP-70 expression as a surrogate for immunoglobulin-variable-region mutations in chronic lymphocytic leukemia. N Engl J Med 348:1764–1775

Cuneo A, Rigolin GM, Bigoni R, De Angeli C, Veronese A, Cavazzini F, Bardi A, Roberti MG, Tammiso E, Agostini P, Ciccone M, Della Porta M, Tieghi A, Cavazzini L, Negrini M, Castoldi G (2004) Chronic lymphocytic leukemia with 6q− shows distinct hematological features and intermediate prognosis. Leukemia 18:476–483

Dalla-Favera R, Migliazza A, Chang CC, Niu H, Pasqualucci L, Butler M, Shen Q, Cattoretti G (1999) Molecular pathogenesis of B cell malignancy: the role of bCL-6. Curr Top Microbiol Immunol 246:257–263

Damle RN, Wasil T, Fais F, Ghiotto F, Valetto A, Allen SL, Buchbinder A, Budman D, Dittmar K, Kolitz J, Lichtman SM, Schulman P, Vinciguerra VP, Rai KR, Ferrarini M, Chiorazzi N (1999) IgV gene mutation status and CD38 expression as novel prognostic indicators in chronic lymphocytic leukemia. Blood 94:1840–1847

Damle RN, Ghiotto F, Valetto A, Albesiano E, Fais F, Yan XJ, Sison CP, Allen SL, Kolitz J, Schulman P, Vinciguerra VP, Budde P, Frey J, Rai KR, Ferrarini M, Chiorazzi N (2002) B-cell chronic lymphocytic leukemia cells express a surface membrane phenotype of activated, antigen-experienced B lymphocytes. Blood 99:4087–4093

Damle RN, Batliwalla FM, Ghiotto F, Valetto A, Albesiano E, Sison C, Allen SL, Kolitz J, Vinciguerra VP, Kudalkar P, Wasil T, Rai KR, Ferrarini M, Gregersen PK, Chiorazzi N (2004) Telomere length and telomerase activity delineate distinctive replicative features of the B-CLL subgroups defined by immunoglobulin V gene mutations. Blood 103:375–382

de Vinuesa CG, Cook MC, Ball J, Drew M, Sunners Y, Cascalho M, Wabl M, Klaus GG, MacLennan IC (2000) Germinal centers without T cells. J Exp Med 191:485–494

Del Poeta G, Maurillo L, Venditti A, Buccisano F, Epiceno AM, Capelli G, Tamburini A, Suppo G, Battaglia A, Del Principe MI, Del Moro B, Masi M, Amadori S (2001) Clinical significance of CD38 expression in chronic lymphocytic leukemia. Blood 98:2633–2639

Dewald GW, Brockman SR, Paternoster SF, Bone ND, O'Fallon JR, Allmer C, James CD, Jelinek DF, Tschumper RC, Hanson CA, Pruthi RK, Witzig TE, Call TG, Kay NE (2003) Chromosome anomalies detected by interphase fluorescence in situ hybridization: correlation with significant biological features of B-cell chronic lymphocytic leukaemia. Br J Haematol 121:287–295

Dohner H, Stilgenbauer S, Benner A, Leupolt E, Krober A, Bullinger L, Dohner K, Bentz M, Lichter P (2000) Genomic aberrations and survival in chronic lymphocytic leukemia. N Engl J Med 343:1910–1916

Economopoulos T, Fotopoulos S, Hatzioannou J, Gardikas C (1982) 'Prolymphocytoid' cells in chronic lymphocytic leukaemia and their prognostic significance. Scand J Haematol 28:238–242

Enno A, Catovsky D, O'Brien M, Cherchi M, Kumaran TO, Galton DA (1979) 'Prolymphocytoid' transformation of chronic lymphocytic leukaemia. Br J Haematol 41:9–18

Fagarasan S, Watanabe N, Honjo T (2000) Generation, expansion, migration and activation of mouse B1 cells. Immunol Rev 176:205–215

Fais F, Ghiotto F, Hashimoto S, Sellars B, Valetto A, Allen SL, Schulman P, Vinciguerra VP, Rai K, Rassenti LZ, Kipps TJ, Dighiero G, Schroeder HW Jr, Ferrarini M, Chiorazzi N (1998) Chronic lymphocytic leukemia B cells express restricted sets of mutated and unmutated antigen receptors. J Clin Invest 102:1515–1525

Fukuda T, Yoshida T, Okada S, Hatano M, Miki T, Ishibashi K, Okabe S, Koseki H, Hirosawa S, Taniguchi M, Miyasaka N, Tokuhisa T (1997) Disruption of the Bcl6 gene results in an impaired germinal center formation. J Exp Med 186:439–448

Geisler CH, Hou-Jensen K, Jensen OM, Tinggaard-Pedersen N, Hansen MM, Hansen NE, Holm M, Christensen BE, Drivsholm A, Nielsen JB, Thorling K, Andersen E, Larsen JK, Anderson PK (1996) The bone-marrow infiltration pattern in B-cell chronic lymphocytic leukemia is not an important prognostic factor. Danish CLL Study Group. Eur J Haematol 57:292–300

Ghia P, Guida G, Stella S, Gottardi D, Geuna M, Strola G, Scielzo C, Caligaris-Cappio F (2003) The pattern of CD38 expression defines a distinct subset of chronic lymphocytic leukemia (CLL) patients at risk of disease progression. Blood 101:1262–1269

Ghiotto F, Fais F, Valetto A, Albesiano E, Hashimoto S, Dono M, Ikematsu H, Allen SL, Kolitz J, Rai KR, Nardini M, Tramontano A, Ferrarini M, Chiorazzi N (2004) Remarkably similar antigen receptors among a subset of patients with chronic lymphocytic leukemia. J Clin Invest 113:1008–1016

Glassman AB, Harper-Allen EA, Hayes KJ, Hopwood VL, Gutterman EE, Zagryn SP (1998) Chromosome 6 abnormalities associated with prolymphocytic acceleration in chronic lymphocytic leukemia. Ann Clin Lab Sci 28:24–29

Goldin LR, Pfeiffer RM, Li X, Hemminki K (2004) Familial risk of lymphoproliferative tumors in families of patients with chronic lymphocytic leukemia: results from the Swedish Family-Cancer Database. Blood 104:1850–1854

Gonzalez H, Maloum K, Remy F, Merle-Beral H, Lesty C (2002) Cleaved lymphocytes in chronic lymphocytic leukemia: a detailed retrospective analysis of diagnostic features. Leuk Lymphoma 43:555–564

Hamblin TJ, Davis Z, Gardiner A, Oscier DG, Stevenson FK (1999) Unmutated Ig V(H) genes are associated with a more aggressive form of chronic lymphocytic leukemia. Blood 94:1848–1854

Hamblin TJ, Orchard JA, Ibbotson RE, Davis Z, Thomas PW, Stevenson FK, Oscier DG (2002) CD38 expression and immunoglobulin variable region mutations are independent prognostic variables in chronic lymphocytic leukemia, but CD38 expression may vary during the course of the disease. Blood 99:1023–1029

Harley CB (1991) Telomere loss: mitotic clock or genetic time bomb? Mutat Res 256:271–282

Hashimoto S, Dono M, Wakai M, Allen SL, Lichtman SM, Schulman P, Vinciguerra VP, Ferrarini M, Silver J, Chiorazzi N (1995) Somatic diversification and selection of immunoglobulin heavy and light chain variable region genes in IgG+ CD5+ chronic lymphocytic leukemia B cells. J Exp Med 181:1507–1517

Haslinger C, Schweifer N, Stilgenbauer S, Dohner H, Lichter P, Kraut N, Stratowa C, Abseher R (2004) Microarray gene expression profiling of B-cell chronic lymphocytic leukemia subgroups defined by genomic aberrations and VH mutation status. J Clin Oncol 22:3937–3949

Heintel D, Schwarzinger I, Chizzali-Bonfadin C, Thalhammer R, Schwarzmeier J, Fritzer-Szekeres M, Weltermann A, Simonitsch I, Lechner K, Jaeger U (2001) Association of CD38 antigen expression with other prognostic parameters in early stages of chronic lymphocytic leukemia. Leuk Lymphoma 42:1315–1321

Hivroz C, Grillot-Courvalin C, Brouet JC, Seligmann M (1986) Heterogeneity of responsiveness of chronic lymphocytic leukemic B cells to B cell growth factor or interleukin 2. Eur J Immunol 16:1001–1004

Hodes RJ (1999) Telomere length, aging, and somatic cell turnover. J Exp Med 190:153–156

Horwitz M, Goode EL, Jarvik GP (1996) Anticipation in familial leukemia. Am J Hum Genet 59:990–998

Huh YO, Pugh WC, Kantarjian HM, Stass SA, Cork A, Trujillo JM, Keating MJ (1994) Cell kinetic analysis of interleukin-2 receptor-tested chronic lymphocytic leukemia using the AgNOR silver stain. Am J Clin Pathol 101:283–289

Hultdin M, Rosenquist R, Thunberg U, Tobin G, Norrback KF, Johnson A, Sundstrom C, Roos G (2003) Association between telomere length and V(H) gene mutation status in chronic lymphocytic leukaemia: clinical and biological implications. Br J Cancer 88:593–598

Ibrahim S, Keating M, Do KA, O'Brien S, Huh YO, Jilani I, Lerner S, Kantarjian HM, Albitar M (2001) CD38 expression as an important prognostic factor in B-cell chronic lymphocytic leukemia. Blood 98:181–186

Ishibe N, Sgambati MT, Fontaine L, Goldin LR, Jain N, Weissman N, Marti GE, Caporaso NE (2001) Clinical characteristics of familial B-CLL in the National Cancer Institute Familial Registry. Leuk Lymphoma 42:99–108

Ishibe N, Prieto D, Hosack DA, Lempicki RA, Goldin LR, Raffeld M, Marti GE, Caporaso NE (2002) Telomere length and heavy-chain mutation status in familial chronic lymphocytic leukemia. Leuk Res 26:791–794

Jelinek DF, Tschumper RC, Geyer SM, Bone ND, Dewald GW, Hanson CA, Stenson MJ, Witzig TE, Tefferi A, Kay NE (2001) Analysis of clonal B-cell CD38 and immunoglobulin variable region sequence status in relation to clinical outcome for B-chronic lymphocytic leukaemia. Br J Haematol 115:854–861

Johnson TA, Rassenti LZ, Kipps TJ (1997) Ig VH1 genes expressed in B cell chronic lymphocytic leukemia exhibit distinctive molecular features. J Immunol 158:235–246

Karray S, Merle-Beral H, Vazquez A, Gerard JP, Debre P, Galanaud P (1987) Functional heterogeneity of B-CLL lymphocytes: dissociated responsiveness to growth factors and distinct requirements for a first activation signal. Blood 70:1105–1110

Kelsoe G (1994) B cell diversification and differentiation in the periphery. J Exp Med 180:5–6

Kipps TJ (1989) The CD5 B cell. Adv Immunol 47:117–185

Kipps TJ, Tomhave E, Pratt LF, Duffy S, Chen PP, Carson DA (1989) Developmentally restricted immunoglobulin heavy chain variable region gene expressed at high frequency in chronic lymphocytic leukemia. Proc Natl Acad Sci U S A 86:5913–5917

Klein U, Tu Y, Stolovitzky GA, Mattioli M, Cattoretti G, Husson H, Freedman A, Inghirami G, Cro L, Baldini L, Neri A, Califano A, Dalla-Favera R (2001) Gene expression profiling of B cell chronic lymphocytic leukemia reveals a homogeneous phenotype related to memory B cells. J Exp Med 194:1625–1638

Krober A, Seiler T, Benner A, Bullinger L, Bruckle E, Lichter P, Dohner H, Stilgenbauer S (2002) V(H) mutation status, CD38 expression level, genomic aberrations, and survival in chronic lymphocytic leukemia. Blood 100:1410–1416

Kroft SH, Finn WG, Kay NE, Peterson LC (1997) Isolated 13q14 abnormalities and normal karyotypes are associated with typical lymphocyte morphology in B-cell chronic lymphocytic leukemia. Am J Clin Pathol 107:275–282

Kusam S, Vasanwala FH, Dent AL (2004) Transcriptional repressor BCL-6 immortalizes germinal center-like B cells in the absence of p53 function. Oncogene 23:839–844

Lanham S, Hamblin T, Oscier D, Ibbotson R, Stevenson F, Packham G (2003) Differential signaling via surface IgM is associated with VH gene mutational status and CD38 expression in chronic lymphocytic leukemia. Blood 101:1087–1093

Lankester AC, van Schijndel GM, van der Schoot CE, van Oers MH, van Noesel CJ, van Lier RA (1995) Antigen receptor nonresponsiveness in chronic lymphocytic leukemia B cells. Blood 86:1090–1097

Lanza F, Moretti S, Latorraca A, Scapoli G, Rigolin F, Castoldi G (1992) Flow cytochemical analysis of peripheral lymphocytes in chronic B-lymphocytic leukemia. Prognostic role of the blast count determined by the H*1 system and its correlation with morphologic features. Leuk Res 16:639–646

Lin K, Manocha S, Harris RJ, Matrai Z, Sherrington PD, Pettitt AR (2003) High frequency of p53 dysfunction and low level of VH mutation in chronic lymphocytic leukemia patients using the VH3-21 gene segment. Blood 102:1145–1146

Ma Y, Mansour A, Bekele BN, Zhou X, Keating MJ, O'Brien S, Giles FJ, Albitar M (2004) The clinical significance of large cells in bone marrow in patients with chronic lymphocytic leukemia. Cancer 100:2167–2175

Mainou-Fowler T, Dignum HM, Proctor SJ, Summerfield GP (2004) The prognostic value of CD38 expression and its quantification in B cell chronic lymphocytic leukemia (B-CLL). Leuk Lymphoma 45:455–462

Marti GE, Zenger V, Caproaso NE, Brown M, Washington GC, Carter P, Schechter G, Noguchi P (1989) Antigenic expression of B-cell chronic lymphocytic leukemic lymphocytes. Anal Quant Cytol Histol 11:315–323

Martin F, Kearney JF (2002) Marginal-zone B cells. Nat Rev Immunol 2:323–335

Matutes E, Polliack A (2000) Morphological and immunophenotypic features of chronic lymphocytic leukemia. Rev Clin Exp Hematol 4:22–47

Matutes E, Oscier D, Garcia-Marco J, Ellis J, Copplestone A, Gillingham R, Hamblin T, Lens D, Swansbury GJ, Catovsky D (1996) Trisomy 12 defines a group of CLL with atypical morphology: correlation between cytogenetic, clinical and laboratory features in 544 patients. Br J Haematol 92:382–388

Mauro FR, De Rossi G, Burgio VL, Caruso R, Giannarelli D, Monarca B, Romani C, Baroni CD, Mandelli F (1994) Prognostic value of bone marrow histology in chronic lymphocytic leukemia. A study of 335 untreated cases from a single institution. Haematologica 79:334–341

Mauro FR, Foa R, Giannarelli D, Cordone I, Crescenzi S, Pescarmona E, Sala R, Cerretti R, Mandelli F (1999) Clinical characteristics and outcome of young chronic lymphocytic leukemia patients: a single institution study of 204 cases. Blood 94:448–454

Mauro FR, Gentile M, Mancini F, Giannarelli D, Guarini A, De Propriis MS, Cerretti R, Foa R (2002) Prognostic significance of lymphocyte morphology in patients with advanced chronic lymphocytic leukemia treated with first line therapy of fludarabine + prednisone. Haematologica 87:602–608

Melo JV, Wardle J, Chetty M, England J, Lewis SM, Galton DA, Catovsky D (1986) The relationship between chronic lymphocytic leukaemia and prolymphocytic leukaemia. III. Evaluation of cell size by morphology and volume measurements. Br J Haematol 64:469–478

Messmer B, Messmer D, Allen SL, Kolitz J, Kudalkar P, Cesar D, Murphy EJ, Koduro P, Ferrarini M, Zupo S, Cutrona G, Damle RN, Wasil T, Rai KR, Hellerstein M:Chiorazzi N (2005) In vivo measurements document the dynamic cellular kinetics of chronic lymphocytic leukemia B cells. J Clin Invest 115:755–764

Messmer BT, Albesiano E, Efremov DG, Ghiotto F, Allen SL, Kolitz J, Foa R, Damle RN, Fais F, Messmer D, Rai KR, Ferrarini M, Chiorazzi N (2004) Multiple distinct sets of stereotyped antigen receptors indicate a role for antigen in promoting chronic lymphocytic leukemia. J Exp Med 200:519–525

Michel F, Merle-Beral H, Legac E, Michel A, Debre P, Bismuth G (1993) Defective calcium response in B-chronic lymphocytic leukemia cells. Alteration of early protein tyrosine phosphorylation and of the mechanism responsible for cell calcium influx. J Immunol 150:3624–3633

Molica S, Alberti A (1987) Prognostic value of the lymphocyte doubling time in chronic lymphocytic leukemia. Cancer 60:2712–2716

Molica S, Alberti A (1988) Investigation of nuclear clefts as a prognostic parameter in chronic lymphocytic leukemia. Eur J Haematol 41:62–65

Molica S, Reverter JC, Alberti A, Montserrat E (1990) Timing of diagnosis and lymphocyte accumulation patterns in chronic lymphocytic leukemia: analysis of their clinical significance. Eur J Haematol 44:277–281

Montserrat E, Sanchez-Bisono J, Vinolas N, Rozman C (1986) Lymphocyte doubling time in chronic lymphocytic leukaemia: analysis of its prognostic significance. Br J Haematol 62:567–575

Montserrat E, Villamor N, Reverter JC, Brugues RM, Tassies D, Bosch F, Aguilar JL, Vives-Corrons JL, Rozman M, Rozma C (1996) Bone marrow assessment in B-cell chronic lymphocytic leukaemia: aspirate or biopsy? A comparative study in 258 patients. Br J Haematol 93:111–116

Mueller LP, Machulla HK (2002) Increased frequency of homozygosity for HLA class II loci in female patients with chronic lymphocytic leukemia. Leuk Lymphoma 43:1013–1019

Neuberger MS, Ehrenstein MR, Klix N, Jolly CJ, Yelamos J, Rada C, Milstein C (1998) Monitoring and interpreting the intrinsic features of somatic hypermutation. Immunol Rev 162:107–116

Niiro H, Clark EA (2002) Regulation of B-cell fate by antigen-receptor signals. Nat Rev Immunol 2:945–956

Orchard JA, Ibbotson RE, Davis Z, Wiestner A, Rosenwald A, Thomas PW, Hamblin TJ, Staudt LM, Oscier DG (2004) ZAP-70 expression and prognosis in chronic lymphocytic leukaemia. Lancet 363:105–111

Orfao A, Gonzalez M, San Miguel JF, Canizo MC, Galindo P, Caballero MD, Jimenez R, Lopez-Borrasca A (1988) Clinical and immunological findings in large B-cell chronic lymphocytic leukemia. Clin Immunol Immunopathol 46:177–185

Orfao A, Ciudad J, Gonzalez M, San Miguel JF, Garcia AR, Lopez-Berges MC, Ramos F, Del Canizo MC, Rios A, Sanz M, et al (1992) Prognostic value of S-phase white blood cell count in B-cell chronic lymphocytic leukemia. Leukemia 6:47–51

Oscier DG, Stevens J, Hamblin TJ, Pickering RM, Lambert R, Fitchett M (1990) Correlation of chromosome abnormalities with laboratory features and clinical course in B-cell chronic lymphocytic leukaemia. Br J Haematol 76:352–358

Oscier DG, Matutes E, Copplestone A, Pickering RM, Chapman R, Gillingham R, Catovsky D, Hamblin TJ (1997a) Atypical lymphocyte morphology: an adverse prognostic factor for disease progression in stage A CLL independent of trisomy 12. Br J Haematol 98:934–939

Oscier DG, Thompsett A, Zhu D, Stevenson FK (1997b) Differential rates of somatic hypermutation in V(H) genes among subsets of chronic lymphocytic leukemia defined by chromosomal abnormalities. Blood 89:4153–4160

Oscier DG, Gardiner AC, Mould SJ, Glide S, Davis ZA, Ibbotson RE, Corcoran MM, Chapman RM, Thomas PW, Copplestone JA, Orchard JA, Hamblin TJ (2002) Multivariate analysis of prognostic factors in CLL: clinical stage, IGVH gene mutational status, and loss or mutation of the p53 gene are independent prognostic factors. Blood 100:1177–1184

Ottaggio L, Viaggi S, Zunino A, Zupo S, Rossi E, Spriano M, Abbondanolo A, Ferraruini M (2003) Chromosome aberrations evaluated by comparative genomic hybridization in B-cell chronic lymphocytic leukemia: correlation with CD38 expression. Haematologica 88:769–777

Pasqualucci L, Migliazza A, Fracchiolla N, William C, Neri A, Baldini L, Chaganti RSK, Klein U, Kuppers R, Rajewsky K, Dalla-Favera R (1998) BCL-6 mutations in normal germinal center B cells: evidence of somatic hypermutation acting outside Ig loci. Proc Natl Acad Sci USA 95:11816–11821

Pasqualucci L, Neri A, Baldini L, Dalla-Favera R, Migliazza A (2000) BCL-6 mutations are associated with immunoglobulin variable heavy chain mutations in B-cell chronic lymphocytic leukemia. Cancer Res 60:5644–5648

Pileri SA, Sabattini E, Agostinelli C, Bodega L, Rossi M, Zinzani PL, Marafioti T (2004) Histopathology of B-cell chronic lymphocytic leukemia. Hematol Oncol Clin North Am 18:807–826

Pritsch O, Troussard X, Magnac C, Mauro FR, Davi F, Payelle-Brogard B, Dumas G, Pulik M, Clerget F, Mandelli F, Chiorazzi N, Schroeder HW Jr, Leporrier M, Dighiero G (1999) VH gene usage by family members affected with chronic lymphocytic leukaemia. Br J Haematol 107:616–624

Que TH, Marco JG, Ellis J, Matutes E, Babapulle VB, Boyle S, Catovsky D (1993) Trisomy 12 in chronic lymphocytic leukemia detected by fluorescence in situ hybridization: analysis by stage, immunophenotype, and morphology. Blood 82:571–575

Ranheim EA, Cantwell MJ, Kipps TJ (1995) Expression of CD27 and its ligand, CD70, on chronic lymphocytic leukemia B cells. Blood 85:3556–3565

Rassenti LZ, Hunynh L, Toy TL, Chen L, Keating MJ, Gribben JG, Neuberg DS, Flinn IW, Rai KR, Byrd JC, Kay NE, Greaves A, Weiss A, Kipps TJ (2004) ZAP-70 compared with immunoglobulin heavy-chain gene mutation status as a predictor of disease progression in chronic lymphocytic leukemia. N Engl J Med 351:893–901

Rosenwald A, Alizadeh AA, Widhopf G, Simon R, Davis RE, Yu X, Yang L, Pickeral OK, Rassenti LZ, Powell J, Botstein D, Byrd JC, Grever MR, Cheson BD, Chiorazzi N, Wilson WH, Kipps TJ, Brown PO, Staudt LM (2001) Relation of gene expression phenotype to immunoglobulin mutation genotype in B cell chronic lymphocytic leukemia. J Exp Med 194:1639–1647

Sahota SS, Davis Z, Hamblin TJ, Stevenson FK (2000) Somatic mutation of bcl-6 genes can occur in the absence of V(H) mutations in chronic lymphocytic leukemia. Blood 95:3534–3540

Sakai A, Marti GE, Caporaso N, Pittaluga S, Touchman JW, Fend F, Raffeld M (2000) Analysis of expressed immunoglobulin heavy chain genes in familial B-CLL. Blood 95:1413–1419

Sarfati M (1993) CD23 and chronic lymphocytic leukemia. Blood Cells 19:591–596

Sarsotti E, Marugan I, Benet I, Terol MJ, Sanchez-Izquierdo D, Tormo M, Rubio-Moscardo F, Martinez-Climent JA, Garcia-Conde J (2004) Bcl-6 mutation status provides clinically valuable information in early-stage B-cell chronic lymphocytic leukemia. Leukemia 18:743–746

Schroeder HW Jr, Dighiero G (1994) The pathogenesis of chronic lymphocytic leukemia: analysis of the antibody repertoire. Immunol Today 15:288–294

Shen HM, Peters A, Baron B, Zhu X, Storb U (1998) Mutation of BCL-6 gene in normal B cells by the process of somatic hypermutation of Ig genes. Science 280:1750–1752

Stevenson F, Caligaris-Cappio F (2004) Chronic lymphocytic leukemia: revelations from the B-cell receptor. Blood 103:4389–4395

Stilgenbauer S, Lichter P, Dohner H (2001) Genomic aberrations in B cell chronic lymphocytic leukemia. In: Cheson BD (ed) Chronic lymphoid leukemias. Marcel Dekker, New York, pp 353–pp 376

Summersgill B, Thornton P, Atkinson S, Matutes E, Shipley J, Catovsky D, Houlston RS, Yuille MR (2002) Chromosomal imbalances in familial chronic lymphocytic leukaemia: a comparative genomic hybridisation analysis. Leukemia 16:1229–1232

Ternynck T, Dighiero G, Follezou J, Binet JL (1974) Comparison of normal and CLL lymphocyte surface Ig determinants using peroxidase-labeled antibodies. I. Detection and quantitation of light chain determinants. Blood 43:789–795

Theodorou I, Abel L, Mauro F, Duprey B, Magnac C, Payelle-Brogard B, Davi F, Dighiero G (2002) High occurrence of DRB1 11 in chronic lymphocytic leukaemia families. Br J Haematol 119:713–715

Tobin G, Thunberg U, Johnson A, Thorn I, Soderberg O, Hultdin M, Botling J, Enblad G, Sallstrom J, Sundstrom C, Roos G, Rosenquist R (2002) Somatically mutated Ig V(H)3-21 genes characterize a new subset of chronic lymphocytic leukemia. Blood 99:2262–2264

Tobin G, Thunberg U, Johnson A, Eriksson I, Soderberg O, Karlsson K, Merup M, Juliusson G, Vilpo J, Enblad G, Sundstrom C, Roos G, Rosenquist R (2003) Chronic lymphocytic leukemias utilizing the VH3-21 gene display highly restricted Vlambda2-14 gene use and homologous CDR3s: implicating recognition of a common antigen epitope. Blood 101:4952–4957

Tobin G, Thunberg U, Karlsson K, Murray F, Laurell A, Willander K, Enblad G, Merup M, Vilpo J, Juliusson G, Sundstrom C, Soderberg O, Roos G, Rosenquist R (2004) Subsets with restricted immunoglobulin gene rearrangement features indicate a role for antigen selection in the development of chronic lymphocytic leukemia. Blood 104:2879–2885

Trentin L, Zambello R, Sancetta R, Facco M, Cerutti A, Perin A, Siviero M, Basso U, Bortolin M, Adami F, Agostini C, Semenzato G (1997) B lymphocytes from patients with chronic lymphoproliferative disorders are equipped with different costimulatory molecules. Cancer Res 57:4940–4947

Vallespi T, Montserrat E, Sanz MA (1991) Chronic lymphocytic leukaemia: prognostic value of lymphocyte morphological subtypes. A multivariate survival analysis in 146 patients. Br J Haematol 77:478–485

van Oers MH, Pals ST, Evers LM, van der Schoot CE, Koopman G, Bonfrer JM, Hintzen RQ, von dem Borne AE, van Lier RA (1993) Expression and release of CD27 in human B-cell malignancies. Blood 82:3430–3436

Vinolas N, Reverter JC, Urbano-Ispizua A, Montserrat E, Rozman C (1987) Lymphocyte doubling time in chronic lymphocytic leukemia: an update of its prognostic significance. Blood Cells 12:457–470

Wakai M, Hashimoto S, Omata M, Sthoeger ZM, Allen SL, Lichtman SM, Schulman P, Vinciguerra VP, Diamond B, Dono M, et al (1994) IgG+, CD5+ human chronic lymphocytic leukemia B cells. Production of IgG antibodies that exhibit diminished autoreactivity and IgG subclass skewing. Autoimmunity 19:39–48

Weller S, Faili A, Garcia C, Braun MC, Le Deist FF, de Saint Basile GG, Hermine O, Fischer A, Reynaud CA, Weill JC (2001) CD40-CD40L independent Ig gene hypermutation suggests a second B cell diversification pathway in humans. Proc Natl Acad Sci U S A 98:1166–1170

Widhopf GF 2nd, Rassenti LZ, Toy TL, Gribben JG, Wierda WG, Kipps TJ (2004) Chronic lymphocytic leukemia B cells of more than 1% of patients express virtually identical immunoglobulins. Blood 104:2499–2504

Wiernik PH, Ashwin M, Hu XP, Paietta E, Brown K (2001) Anticipation in familial chronic lymphocytic leukaemia. Br J Haematol 113:407–414

Wiestner A, Rosenwald A, Barry TS, Wright G, Davis RE, Henrickson SE, Zhao H, Ibbotson RE, Orchard JA, Davis Z, Stetler-Stevenson M, Raffeld M, Arthur DC, Marti GE, Wilson WH, Hamblin TJ, Oscier DG, Staudt LM (2003) ZAP-70 expression identifies a chronic lymphocytic leukemia subtype with unmutated immunoglobulin genes, inferior clinical outcome, and distinct gene expression profile. Blood 101:4944–4951

Yuille MR, Houlston RS, Catovsky D (1998) Anticipation in familial chronic lymphocytic leukaemia. Leukemia 12:1696–1698

Yuille MR, Condie A, Hudson CD, Bradshaw PS, Stone EM, Matutes E, Catovsky D, Houlston RS (2002) ATM mutations are rare in familial chronic lymphocytic leukemia. Blood 100:603–609

Zupo S, Isnardi L, Megna M, Massara R, Malavasi F, Dono M, Cosulich E, Ferrarini M (1996) CD38 expression distinguishes two groups of B-cell chronic lymphocytic leukemias with different responses to anti-IgM antibodies and propensity to apoptosis. Blood 88:1365–1374

CTMI (2005) 294:135–145

Differential Effects on CLL Cell Survival Exerted by Different Microenvironmental Elements

P. Ghia[1] (✉) · P. Circosta[2] · C. Scielzo[1] · A. Vallario[2] · A. Camporeale[1] · L. Granziero[2] · F. Caligaris-Cappio[1]

[1]Department of Oncology, Università Vita-Salute, San Raffaele, Via Olgettina 60, 20132 Milano, Italy
ghia.paolo@hsr.it

[2]Department of Oncological Sciences, University of Torino, Laboratory of Cancer Immunology, Institute for Cancer Research and Treatment, Strada Provinciale 142, 10060 Candiolo (TO), Italy

Abstract Selected microenvironmental stimuli confer to leukemic cells a growth advantage and an extended survival. We aimed at dissecting the differential support provided by the different cellular components of the microenvironment where CLL cells accumulate. To this end we cultured purified CLL cells in vitro in the presence or absence of different accessory cells (stromal cells, autologous T lymphocytes) and/or soluble molecules (IL-4, sCD40L) and assessed the leukemic cell response in terms of cell viability and chemoattracting capacity. The results indicate that both T lymphocytes and stromal cells are involved in sustaining the survival of leukemic B cells, but indicate that their support is different in terms of time of onset and duration. T cells have a short-term support activity while stromal cells provide long-term support.

Abbreviations

APC	Allophycocyanin
CD40-NR	CD40-non-responders
CD40-R	CD40-responder
FITC	Fluorescein isothiocyanate
IL-4	Interleukin 4
PE	Phycoerythrin
sCD40L	Soluble CD40 Ligand

1 Introduction

Chronic lymphocytic leukemia (CLL) is regarded as the prototype of chronic lymphoproliferative disorders, as it recapitulates many of the common features of these disorders. CLL is characterized by a relentless accumulation of monoclonal $CD5^+$ B lymphocytes, which appear to be strictly dependent on the surrounding microenvironment, at least in the initial phases of the disease. CLL cells maintain their capacity to respond to selected external stimuli that confer to leukemic cells a growth advantage and an extended survival. Accordingly, both cellular and soluble components of the environments infiltrated by leukemic cells have been shown to participate in progression of the disease [1]. In particular, stromal cells have the capacity to sustain prolonged viability of the leukemic clone when it is placed in vitro for culture [2, 3]. In addition, peripheral blood (PB) obtained from CLL patients contains cells that can differentiate into adherent nurse-like cells that appear to be able to protect leukemic cells from spontaneous apoptosis [4].

It is also known that normal activated $CD3^+$ $CD4^+$ $CD40L^+$ T cells are detected in CLL-involved tissues [5, 6], mainly gathering in the so-called pseudo-follicles (PF), where leukemic cells have a blast-like phenotype and show distinct biological features such as intense proliferative activity and specific chemokine production [6, 7]. All these features are reminiscent of a T cell-mediated type of activation occurring in vivo. In keeping with this possibility, several reports indicate that CD40/CD40L interactions play a relevant pathogenetic role. CD40 stimulation can rescue CLL cells from apoptosis and induce their proliferation and activation as witnessed by the upregulation of several molecules (e.g., CD80, CD95) on the cell surface and the induction of chemokine production (e.g., CCL-22/MDC, CCL-17/TARC) [6, 8–13]. Nevertheless, not all CLL clones respond to in vitro CD40 stimulation, indicating the existence of a CLL subset of CD40L-non-responders [6, 7, 11].

Taken together, these observations lead to the view that bystander/malignant cell contacts deliver signals important for maintenance and expansion of leukemic B cells. In addition, as CLL cells secrete chemokines, they can actively shape the microenvironment according to their need by attracting the relevant bystander accessory cells, which could in turn provide "useful" signals for the expansion of the leukemic clone.

Starting from the concept of the microenvironment/malignant clone interplay, we aimed at dissecting the differential support provided by the different cellular components present within the infiltrated tissues. To this end, we cultured purified CLL cells in vitro in the presence or absence of different accessory cells (i.e., stromal cells, T lymphocytes) and/or soluble molecules (i.e., IL-4, sCD40L), and assessed the capacity of leukemic cells to respond in terms of cell viability and chemoattracting capacity. The results led us to present a model that highlights the role of both T lymphocytes and stromal cells in sustaining the survival of leukemic B cells, though it appears that the kind of support provided by the two cell types diverges in terms of onset and duration. Our findings allowed us to ascribe to T cells a short-term support activity as compared to a long-term support, provided by stromal cells.

2 Materials and Methods

2.1 Cells and Purification

Leukemic lymphocytes were obtained from the peripheral blood of 12 consecutive, unselected CLL patients, diagnosed according to the National Cancer Institute-Working Group (NCI-WG) [14]. All patients were untreated (7 cases) or off-therapy (5 cases) for more than 6 months. After centrifugation through a Ficoll-Hypaque (FH) density gradient, mononuclear cells were further purified by negative depletion after labeling with a mixture of anti-CD14, -CD16, -CD56, and -CD11c (Caltag Laboratories) monoclonal antibodies and separation on magnetic-activated cell separation (MACS) column, according to the manufacturer's instruction. The enriched fraction was then incubated with anti-CD7 antibody (Caltag Laboratories), and separated on MACS column in order to obtain leukemic $CD19^+$ B cells (negative fraction) and normal $CD3^+$ T cells (positive fraction). Leukemic $CD19^+$ cells and $CD3^+$ T cells were always more than 97% pure, as detected by cytofluorograph analysis (see Sect. 2.3).

Purified $CD3^+$ T cells were activated in vitro by concomitant stimulation with anti-CD3- and anti-CD28-coated plates [7].

Stromal cell lines HS5 and HS27A were purchased from ATCC–LGC Promochem (SW London, UK), and maintained in RPMI 1640 medium supplemented with 10% fetal calf serum (FCS), 2 mM L-glutamine, and 15 µg/ml gentamicin (complete RPMI–cRPMI) (Invitrogen-Lifetechnologies, Glasgow, UK). In two CLL patients, stromal cells were obtained from autologous bone marrow mononuclear cells, as previously described [7], isolated on a FH density gradient, and cultured in α-minimal essential medium (α-MEM; Invitrogen-Life Technologies, Glasgow, UK) supplemented with 20% FCS and 2×10–6 M methylprednisolone (Sigma-Aldrich, Milano, Italy). The adherent cells were weekly fed, by replacing 50% of the medium until confluent layers were visible.

2.2 Cell Culture

Purified leukemic $CD19^+CD5^+$ B cells, $CD3^+$ T cells and stromal cells were cultured in vitro in cRPMI at the following conditions:

- Purified leukemic $CD19^+CD5^+$ B cells in medium alone
- Purified $CD3^+$ T cells in medium alone
- Activated $CD3^+$ T cells in medium alone
- Purified leukemic B cells in the presence of soluble human CD40L (sCD40L) at either 100 ng/ml or 1 µg/ml plus 1 µg/ml of enhancer, according to manufacturer's instructions (Alexis Corporation, San Diego, CA) +/– interleukin 4 (IL-4) (10 ng/ml)
- Purified leukemic B cells in the presence of resting T cells (1:3 ratio)
- Purified leukemic B cells in the presence of activated T cells (1:3 ratio)
- Purified leukemic B cells in the presence of either autologous or immortalized stromal cells

Cultured cells were collected at different time points and further analyzed for phenotypic characterization, apoptosis assessment, or RNA extraction.

Culture supernatants were also collected after 72 h of culture, filtered, frozen, and stored at –80°C for the enzyme-linked immunosorbent assay (ELISA) tests.

2.3 Cytofluorograph Analysis

Three color immunofluorescence analyses were performed, as previously described [15], to identify leukemic cells, to assess the percentage of relevant subpopulations after magnetic depletion and activation after in vitro culture. We used specific antibodies conjugated with fluorescein isothiocyanate (FITC), phycoerythrin (PE) or allophycocyanin (APC): anti-CD3, anti-CD4, anti-CD8, anti-CD95, anti-CD16, anti-CD14 (Caltag Laboratories, San Francisco, CA), anti-CD5, anti-CD80 (BD Biosciences, San Jose, CA), anti-CD19, and anti-CD56 (Beckman-Coulter). Cells were collected at different time points during in vitro culture, as shown in the Results section. For each sample, at least 10,000 events were acquired on a FACSCalibur equipped with a 488 argon ion laser and 635 red diode laser (Becton and Dickinson, San Jose, CA) and analyzed with the CellQuest software system (Becton and Dickinson).

Viability of the cultured cells was assessed with an annexin V-based apoptosis detection kit (R&D Systems, Minneapolis, MN), according to manufacturer's instructions, allowing quantification of early apoptotic cells through detection of phosphatidylserine exposition on cell membrane. At different time points, cells were collected and labeled with PE-conjugated anti-CD19 or with a mixture of PE-labeled anti-CD3, anti-CD16, and anti-CD56 in order to identify leukemic B cells and further incubated with saturating concentrations of annexin V-FITC for 15–30 min at room temperature. Cells were then immediately analyzed on a FACSCalibur.

2.4 RNA Extraction, RT-PCR

Total RNA from cells collected after 24 h of culture was extracted using TRIzol (Invitrogen Life Technologies, Paisley, UK), following the manufacturer's instructions. cDNAs synthesis and polymerase chain reaction (PCR) amplifications for CCL21/MDC, CCL17/TARC, and β-actin were carried out as described previously [6].

2.5 ELISA Assays

The production of the chemokines CCL17/TARC and CCL22/MDC was quantified by ELISA, on day 3 supernatants, using commercially available kits (R&D Systems, Minneapolis, MN). The lower limit of detection of the ELISA was 0.007 ng/ml for CCL17, and 0.0625 ng/ml for CCL22.

3
Results and Discussion

We planned to compare the response of leukemic cells obtained from CLL patients in terms of in vitro viability when exposed to different accessory cells, specifically to stromal cells and resting and activated autologous T lymphocytes. To mimic T cell help, leukemic cells were cultured also in the presence or absence of sCD40L. As previously reported [6, 7, 11], CLL cases could be grouped into CD40-responders (CD40-R) and CD40-non-responders (CD40-NR) according to their in vitro response to CD40L-stimulation. In detail, patients (8/12) whose cells (1) showed induction/upregulation of CD95 and/or CD80, (2) improved their in vitro viability, (3) displayed an induction of a RT-PCR band specific for the chemokines CCL22/MDC and CCL17/TARC, and (4) secreted CCL22/MDC in the supernatants, were defined CD40-R. In contrast, patients (4/12 cases) whose cells showed no phenotypic nor functional modifications after in vitro CD40 stimulation or marginal changes in only one of the four assays (in one case the presence of a PCR band for TARC, in another one CD95 up-regulation) were considered as CD40-NR. Such a behavioral difference was evident also after incubating cells with a 10× concentration of sCD40L (1 μg/ml) (Fig. 1A), used in the hypothesis that the difference might be ascribed to the strength of the signal delivered. CCL22/MDC became detectable also in the supernatants of CD40-NR (mean concentration 2.4 ng/ml), but an eightfold difference in terms of production was evident in CD40-R (mean concentration 18.8 ng/ml) (Fig. 1A).

Both CD40-R and CD40-NR were unable to secrete CCL-17/TARC, though CD40-R cases were successfully induced to express CCL-17/TARC-specific mRNA [6]. The increase of sCD40L concentration slightly modified the pat-

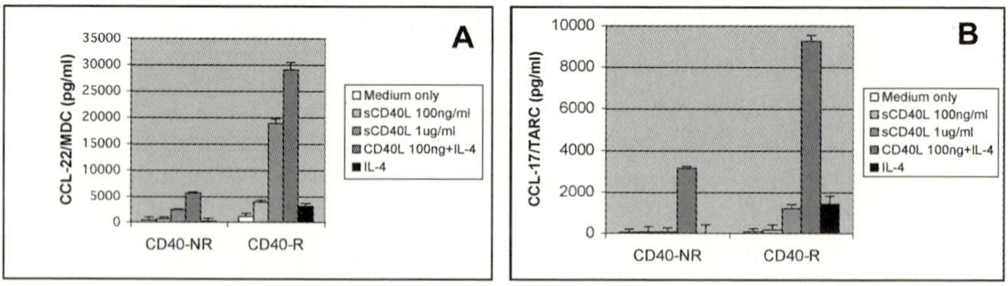

Fig. 1A, B Chemokine production by CLL cells. Supernatants from CLL cells cultured in vitro for 3 days in medium only, in the presence of sCD40L at 100 ng/ml or at 1 μg/ml, of sCD40L 100 ng/ml+IL-4 (10 ng/ml), and IL-4 alone (10 ng/ml) were ELISA tested for the presence of CCL-22/MDC (**A**) and CCL-17/TARC (**B**). Mean values +/− standard errors of 12 cases (3 replicates each) are shown. CD40R and CD40-NR: CD40 responder cases (8) and CD40 non-responder cases (4), respectively tern of secretion, with barely detectable levels produced by CD40-NR (mean concentration 0.03 ng/ml) and minimal quantities released by CD40-R (mean concentration 1.2 ng/ml), (Fig. 1B). As it was previously reported that the combination of T helper (Th)2 cytokines (e.g., IL-4, IL-13, TNF-α) [16, 17] might be able to promote TARC protein secretion from epithelial cells, we added the T cell-produced cytokine IL-4 to our culture system and checked for TARC production in the cell supernatants after 3 days of culture. Of interest, this combination was indeed able to induce the secretion of relevant amounts of TARC (Fig. 1B) in the supernatants of both the CD40-R and the CD40-NR patients. Nevertheless, CD40-R cells produced almost three times the amount released by CD40-NR (mean concentration 9.2 ng/ml vs 3.1 ng/ml) (Fig. 1B). IL-4 alone was able to induce only minimal TARC production from CD40-R cells (mean concentration 1.1 ng/ml) as compared to the sCD40L/IL-4 combination. No secretion was evident in CD40-NR cases cultured in the presence of only IL-4.

While these experimental data underscore the existence of different levels of sensitivity of leukemic cells to different microenvironmental signals, they together concur to the idea that all leukemic cells may indeed respond to external signals if delivered in the proper way and time. This is shown by our experimental approach that tries to reproduce in vitro what is likely to happen in vivo where several signals may act concomitantly or in succession. The implication is that such a differential response may explain the differential behavior of different CLL subtypes where the survival and progressive accumulation of leukemic cells have different dynamics.

Following this line of reasoning, we cultured our CLL samples in the presence of two of the potential players present in the leukemic microenvironment: stromal cells and T lymphocytes. We took advantage of the immortalized human bone marrow cell lines available and, in two selected cases, of primary stromal cells obtained from patients' marrow aspirates [7].

We evaluated the viability of leukemic cells in these different co-culture conditions, at different time points, for up to 2 weeks of culture. As expected [11], CD40-R cells (Fig. 2A and B), but not CD40-NR ones (Fig. 2C and D), showed a better survival in vitro when exposed to sCD40L. Somehow expected was the fact that such a difference in viability was also evident when cells were co-cultured with activated autologous T cells (Fig. 2A–D), in contrast to resting T cells. The sustained viability of leukemic cells in both conditions was apparent during the first week of culture, declining afterwards, due to a progressive onset of apoptosis (short-term survival). Interestingly enough, CLL leukemic cells cultured in the presence of activated T cells showed a faster decline in terms of viability after the first 7 days, when compared to the cells cultured in the presence of sCD40L alone (Fig. 2 A-B). This massive in vitro

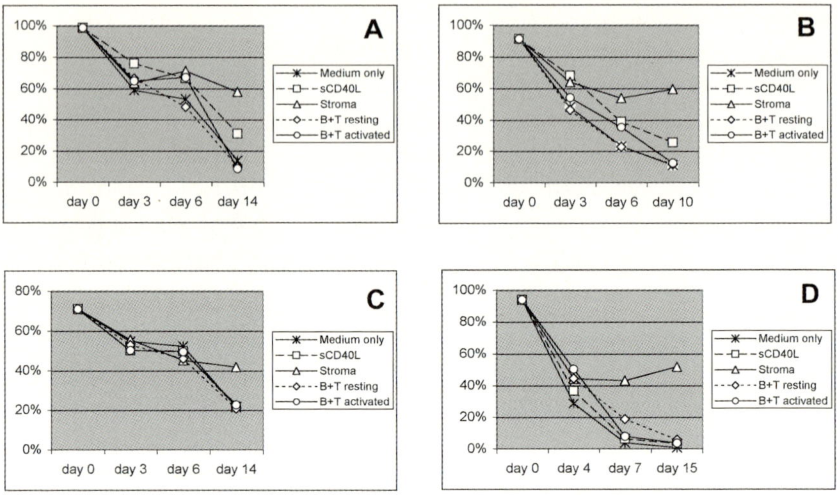

Fig. 2A–D Viability of CLL cells in different co-culture conditions. Time-course experiments of two representative CD40-responder patients (**A**, **B**) and two CD40-non-responders patients (**C**, **D**) whose cells were cultured in medium only, in the presence of sCD40L (100 ng/ml), stromal cells (*stroma*), resting autologous T cells (*B+T resting*) and activated autologous T cells (*B+T activated*). Viability was assessed by cytofluorimetric analysis of annexin V staining and expressed as percentage of viable cells, at the indicated time points

cell death may be likely explained by the fact that T cells after activation will eventually express death-inducing molecules (e.g., CD95L) [18], and during the same period of time CLL cells, after an initial protection, progressively increase their sensitivity to CD95-mediated death [19].

In contrast, by the end of the first week of culture an increase in survival of leukemic cells became evident in the cultures with stromal cells, for both CD40-R and CD40-NR cases (Fig. 2A–D). From that moment on, the number of viable leukemic cells remained stable during the whole culture time (long term survival) of 2 weeks.

According to these data, one can envision a scenario (Fig. 3) where CLL cells infiltrating lymphoid tissues interact with activated T cells, which can be attracted into CLL cells' proximity via CCL22/MDC and CCL-17/TARC production. Leukemic cells will be thus exposed to several cellular or soluble stimuli (e.g., CD40L, IL-4) that can favor their expansion and survival. However, such a nurturing relationship has to come to an end sooner or later as activated T cells carry the potential to limit the progressive expansion of B cells (e.g., via CD95–CD95L interactions), likely leading to a deadly out-

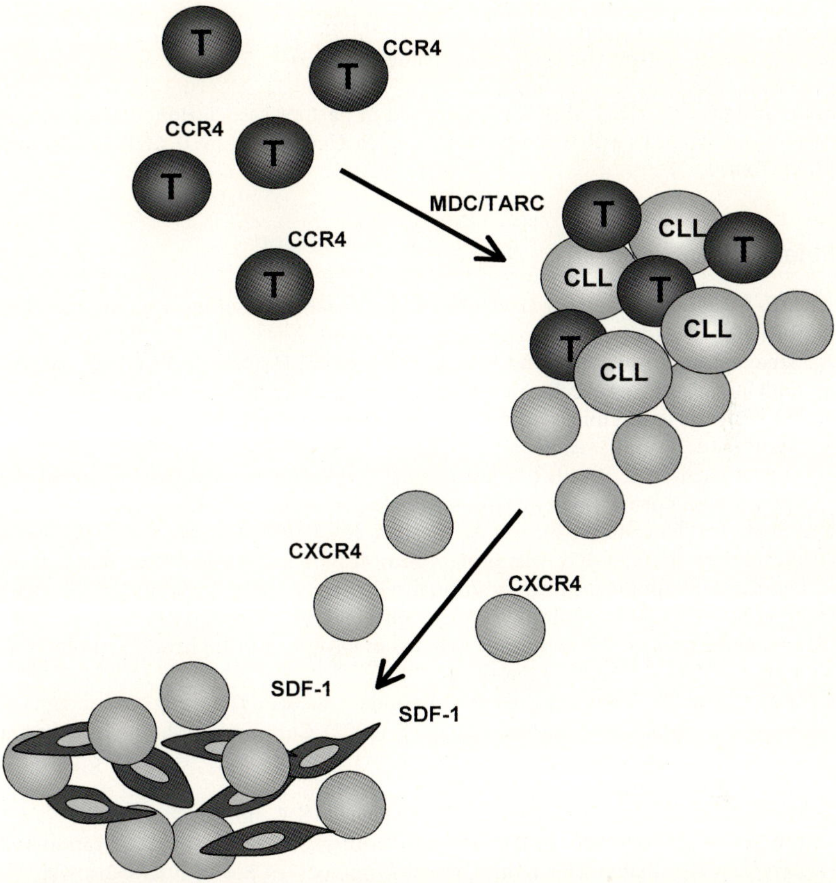

Fig. 3 Hypothetical model of the cellular interplay occurring in the CLL-infiltrated lymphoid tissues. Activated T cells (*dark gray circles*) would be attracted by CLL cells (*light gray circles*) producing CCL22/MDC and CCL17/TARC, binding to the specific CCR4 receptor. CLL cells would be stimulated to proliferate (*large gray circles*) and survive for a short period of time (short-term survival). CLL would then be drifted away from T cells via SDF-1/CXCR4 interactions by the stromal cells that will support long-term survival of leukemic cells

come [19]. As CLL cells express CXCR4 [20], they can be drifted away from T cells towards the surrounding stromal cells, which are the main producers of CXCL12/SDF-1 [21], the CXCR4-specific ligand. Without T cell-mediated activation, leukemic B cells will stop proliferating and producing T cell-attracting chemokines (i.e., CCL22/MDC and CCL17/TARC) [6] and will take advantage of the long-term support mediated by the stromal cells, thereby progressively accumulating within the lymphoid tissues (Fig. 3).

Acknowledgements This work was supported in part by Associazione Italiana per la Ricerca sul Cancro (AIRC), Progetto Strategico Oncologia (PSO) CNR-MIUR, and MURST 40%.

References

1. Ghia P, Caligaris-Cappio F (2000) The indispensable role of microenvironment in the natural history of low-grade B-cell neoplasms. Adv Cancer Res 79:157–173
2. Panayiotidis P, Jones D, Ganeshaguru K, Foroni L, Hoffbrand AV (1996) Human bone marrow stromal cells prevent apoptosis and support the survival of chronic lymphocytic leukaemia cells in vitro. Br J Haematol 92:97–103
3. Lagneaux L, Delforge A, Bron D, De Bruyn C, Stryckmans P (1998) Chronic lymphocytic leukemic B cells but not normal B cells are rescued from apoptosis by contact with normal bone marrow stromal cells. Blood 91:2387–2396
4. Burger JA, Tsukada N, Burger M, Zvaifler NJ, Dell'Aquila M, Kipps TJ (2000) Blood-derived nurse-like cells protect chronic lymphocytic leukemia B cells from spontaneous apoptosis through stromal cell-derived factor-1. Blood 96:2655–2663
5. Pizzolo G, Chilosi M, Ambrosetti A, Semenzato G, Fiore-Donati L, Perona G (1983) Immunohistologic study of bone marrow involvement in B-chronic lymphocytic leukemia. Blood 62:1289–1296
6. Ghia P, Strola G, Granziero L, Geuna M, Guida G, Sallusto F, Ruffing N, Montagna L, Piccoli P, Chilosi M, Caligaris-Cappio F (2002) Chronic lymphocytic leukemia B cells are endowed with the capacity to attract CD4+, CD40L+ T cells by producing CCL22. Eur J Immunol 32:1403–1413
7. Granziero L, Circosta P, Scielzo C, Frisaldi E, Stella S, Geuna M, Giordano S, Ghia P, Caligaris-Cappio F (2003) CD100/Plexin-B1 interactions sustain proliferation and survival of normal and leukemic CD5+ B lymphocytes. Blood 101:1962–1969
8. Wang D, Freeman GJ, Levine H, Ritz J, Robertson MJ (1997) Role of the CD40 and CD95 (APO-1/Fas) antigens in the apoptosis of human B-cell malignancies. Br J Haematol 97:409–417
9. Buske C, Gogowski G, Schreiber K, Rave-Frank M, Hiddemann W, Wormann B (1997) Stimulation of B-chronic lymphocytic leukemia cells by murine fibroblasts, IL-4, anti-CD40 antibodies, and the soluble CD40 ligand. Exp Hematol 25:329–337
10. Kitada S, Zapata JM, Andreeff M, Reed JC (1999) Bryostatin and CD40-ligand enhance apoptosis resistance and induce expression of cell survival genes in B-cell chronic lymphocytic leukaemia. Br J Haematol 106:995–1004
11. Granziero L, Ghia P, Circosta P, Gottardi D, Strola G, Geuna M, Montagna L, Piccoli P, Chilosi M, Caligaris-Cappio F (2001) Survivin is expressed on CD40 stimulation and interfaces proliferation and apoptosis in B-cell chronic lymphocytic leukemia. Blood 97:2777–2783
12. Ranheim EA, Kipps TJ (1993) Activated T cells induce expression of B7/BB1 on normal or leukemic B cells through a CD40-dependent signal. J Exp Med 177:925–935

13. Yellin MJ, Sinning J, Covey LR, Sherman W, Lee JJ, Glickman-Nir E, Sippel KC, Rogers J, Cleary AM, Parker M, et al (1994) T lymphocyte T cell-B cell-activating molecule/CD40-L molecules induce normal B cells or chronic lymphocytic leukemia B cells to express CD80 (B7/BB-1) and enhance their costimulatory activity. J Immunol 153:666–674
14. Cheson BD, Bennett JM, Grever M, Kay N, Keating MJ, O'Brien S, Rai KR (1996) National Cancer Institute-sponsored Working Group guidelines for chronic lymphocytic leukemia: revised guidelines for diagnosis and treatment. Blood 87:4990–4997
15. Ghia P, Guida G, Stella S, Gottardi D, Geuna M, Strola G, Scielzo C, Caligaris-Cappio F (2003) The pattern of CD38 expression defines a distinct subset of chronic lymphocytic leukemia (CLL) patients at risk of disease progression. Blood 101:1262–1269
16. Sekiya T, Miyamasu M, Imanishi M, Yamada H, Nakajima T, Yamaguchi M, Fujisawa T, Pawankar R, Sano Y, Ohta K, Ishii A, Morita Y, Yamamoto K, Matsushima K, Yoshie O, Hirai K (2000) Inducible expression of a Th2-type CC chemokine thymus- and activation-regulated chemokine by human bronchial epithelial cells. J Immunol 165:2205–2213
17. Xiao T, Fujita H, Saeki H, Mitsui H, Sugaya M, Tada Y, Kakinuma T, Torii H, Nakamura K, Asahina A, Tamaki K (2003) Thymus and activation-regulated chemokine (TARC/CCL17) produced by mouse epidermal Langerhans cells is upregulated by TNF-alpha and IL-4 and downregulated by IFN-gamma. Cytokine 23:126–132
18. Nagata S, Golstein P (1995) The Fas death factor. Science 267:1449–1456
19. Chu P, Deforce D, Pedersen IM, Kim Y, Kitada S, Reed JC, Kipps TJ (2002) Latent sensitivity to Fas-mediated apoptosis after CD40 ligation may explain activity of CD154 gene therapy in chronic lymphocytic leukemia. Proc Natl Acad Sci USA 99:3854–3859
20. Burger JA, Burger M, Kipps TJ (1999) Chronic lymphocytic leukemia B cells express functional CXCR4 chemokine receptors that mediate spontaneous migration beneath bone marrow stromal cells. Blood 94:3658–3667
21. Bleul CC, Fuhlbrigge RC, Casasnovas JM, Aiuti A, Springer TA (1996) A highly efficacious lymphocyte chemoattractant, stromal cell-derived factor 1 (SDF-1). J Exp Med 184:1101–1109

CTMI (2005) 294:147–164

Genotypic Prognostic Markers

S. Stilgenbauer (✉) · H. Döhner

Department of Internal Medicine III, University of Ulm, Robert-Koch-Str. 8, Ulm, Germany
stephan.stilgenbauer@medizin.uni-ulm.de

Abstract In chronic lymphocytic leukemia (CLL), genetic analyses by fluorescence in situ hybridization (FISH) and DNA sequencing have greatly improved our understanding of pathogenic events and prognostic markers. On the one hand, there are genomic aberrations, which are detected in over 80% of CLL cases, and genes potentially involved in pathogenesis were identified with ATM in a subset of cases with 11q deletion and p53 in cases with 17p13 deletion. Genetic subgroups with distinct clinical features have been identified, such as the 11q deletion that is associated with marked lymphadenopathy and rapid disease progression, while the 17p deletion predicts treatment failure with alkylating agents as well as fludarabine and short survival times. On the other hand, there is the mutation status of the VH genes that allows the separation of patients into long (mutated *VH*) or short (unmutated *VH*) survival times. V-gene usage, VDJ structure, and gene expression differences in the two subgroups allow insights into differential pathogenic mechanisms and provide further prognostic information (V3-21 usage, ZAP-70 expression). Most importantly, the *VH* mutation status and genomic abnormalities have been shown to be of independent prognostic value in multivariate analysis, appear to allow outcome predication irrespective of the clinical stage, and may therefore allow a risk assessment of individual patients early in the course of the disease.

1 Introduction

Chronic lymphocytic leukemia (CLL) follows an extremely variable clinical course with survival times ranging from months to decades (Zwiebel and Cheson 1998). CLL affects mainly people of advanced age, but about 20% of patients are less than 55 years old. Treatment of early-stage patients with chlorambucil irrespective of risk stratification has not been shown to prolong survival (Dighiero 1998). Therefore, therapeutic procedures had been aimed at palliation, but over recent years, highly effective and potentially curative approaches such as combined antibody-chemotherapy and autologous or allogeneic stem cell transplantation have been developed. The therapeutic options vary markedly with regard to efficacy, toxicity, and cost. In addition, in the light of the broad therapeutic spectrum available, a risk-vs-benefit evaluation based on individual disease characteristics would be desirable. In parallel, there has been dramatic progress in our understanding of pathogenesis and outcome prediction. The standard clinical procedures to estimate prognosis are the clinical staging systems developed by Rai and Binet (Rai 1975; Binet 1981). These systems define early (Rai 0, Binet A), intermediate (Rai I/II, Binet B), and advanced (Rai III/IV, Binet C) stage disease with median estimated survival times of >10, 5–7, and 1–3 years, respectively. However, there is heterogeneity in the course of the disease among individual patients within a single stage group, and, most importantly, the clinical staging systems do not allow us to predict if and at what rate there will be disease progression in an individual patient diagnosed with early-stage disease. To refine outcome prediction for individual patients, there has been intensive work done on additional clinical and biological factors of potential prognostic relevance such as age, gender, and performance status; lymphocyte count, lactate dehydrogenase (LDH) elevation, bone marrow infiltration pattern, or lymphocyte doubling time; soluble CD23, β2-microglobuline (β2-MG), or thymidine kinase (TK); genomic aberrations, gene abnormalities (*p53* and *ATM*), the mutation status of the variable segments of immunoglobulin heavy chain genes (*VH*), or surrogate markers for these factors (CD38, ZAP-70, LPL, etc.) (Damle 1999; Hamblin 1999; Döhner 2000; Kröber 2002; Oscier 2002; Lin 2002; Crespo 2003; Orchard 2003; Dewald 2003; Vasconcelos 2003; Rozman 1984; Montserrat 1986; Di Giovanni 1989; Hallek 1999). Among these factors of potential pathogenic and prognostic relevance, the genetic characteristics of the CLL cells have attained considerable importance. Molecular genetics of CLL can be divided into two major issues: (1) genomic aberrations which may be involved in the initiation and progression of the disease, and (2) the mutation status of the variable segments of VH genes, which may be related to the cellular origin of CLL.

2 Genotypic Prognostic Factors in CLL

2.1 *VH* Mutation Status and Surrogate Markers

Somatically mutated VH genes can be observed in about half of all CLL cases, and a separation was made into two different groups: one with unmutated VH genes, assumed to originate from pregerminal center cells, and another with mutated VH genes, thought to originate from postgerminal center cells (Damle 1999; Hamblin 1999). However, genome-wide gene expression profiling studies revealed a surprisingly homogeneous pattern of gene expression in both subtypes of CLL with only a limited set of genes being differentially expressed in the subgroups (Rosenwald 2001; Klein 2001). Most importantly, it could be demonstrated that the *VH* mutation status is clinically highly relevant (Damle 1999; Hamblin 1999). While CLL with unmutated *VH* shows an unfavorable course with rapid progression, CLL with mutated *VH* often shows slow progression and long survival. Figure 1 shows the survival curves for patients distributed over all stages (n=300) and separately for patients diagnosed with Binet stage A disease (n=189) from the largest published cohort (Kröber 2002). Furthermore, and independently of the mutation status, the usage of specific VH genes such as V3-21 may be associated with an inferior outcome (Tobin 2002).

Due to the technical difficulties in *VH* sequencing, surrogate markers available in a routine hematology laboratory were identified. A correlation

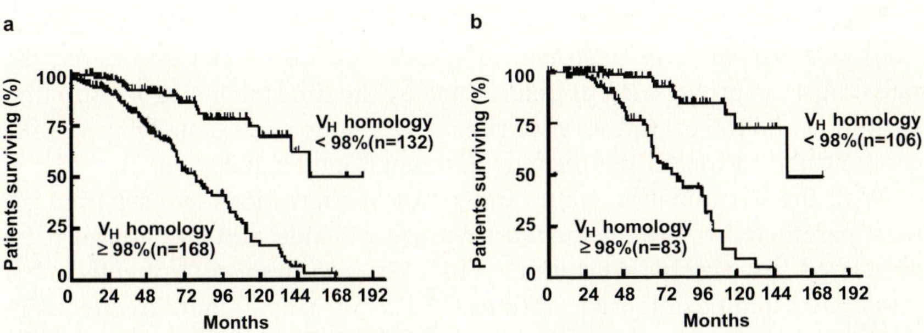

Fig. 1a, b Probability of survival from the date of diagnosis among patients with mutated (*VH* homology<98%) and unmutated (*VH* homology≥98%) *VH* status (Kröber 2002). **a** The estimated median survival times for the *VH* homology≥98 and <98% groups were 79 months and 152 months, respectively. **b** When only patients diagnosed at Binet stage A were evaluated, the estimated median survival times for the *VH* homology≥98% and *VH* homology<98% groups were 79 months vs 152 months was observed between the *VH* mutation status and CD38 expression of the CLL cells, pointing to CD38 expression as a prognostic marker (Damle 1999). Based on genome-wide gene expression studies, other surrogate markers such as ZAP-70 expression were identified and validated (Rosenwald 2000; Crespo 2003). ZAP-70 expression appears to strongly correlate with *VH* mutation status and was therefore a strong prognostic marker in a pivotal study (Crespo 2003). However, for both CD38 and ZAP-70, subsequent studies have yielded controversial results and technical difficulties have emerged: Discordant results have been obtained in different laboratories (for both CD38 and ZAP-70), the expression level may change over time (for CD38), a careful separation of T cells is necessary (for ZAP-70), different cut-off values to distinguish "positive" from "negative" cases were defined (for CD38 and ZAP-70), and approximately 10%–30% of cases show discordant status for CD38 or ZAP-70 as compared to VH in all series described (Hamblin 2002; Kröber 2002; Crespo 2003; Orchard 2003; Ghia 2003).

2.2 Genomic Aberrations and Their Relation to *VH* Mutation Status

The other genetic parameter shown to be of pathogenic and clinical relevance in CLL are genomic aberrations. Genomic aberrations can be identified in about 80% of CLL cases by fluorescence in situ hybridization (FISH) of interphase cell nuclei ("interphase-cytogenetics") with a disease-specific comprehensive probe set (Döhner 2000). Genomic aberrations provide insights into the pathogenesis of the disease since they point to loci of candidate genes (17p13: *p53*; 11q22-q23: *ATM*) and identify subgroups of patients with distinct clinical presentation such as marked lymphadenopathy (11q deletion) and resistance to treatment (17p deletion, see below). Moreover, the rate of disease progression as determined by the time form diagnosis to first treatment and the overall survival time of CLL subgroups defined by specific genomic aberrations is significantly different (Döhner 2000; Fig. 2).

With the *VH* mutation status and genomic aberrations two separate genetic parameters of prognostic relevance are available, and they appear to be correlated. Unfavorable aberrations ($11q^-$, $17p^-$) occur more frequently in *VH* unmutated, and favorable aberrations ($13q^-$, $13q^-$ single) more frequently in the *VH* mutated subgroup (Table 1) (Kröber 2002; Osier 2002; Lin 2002). This unbalanced distribution of genomic aberrations emphasizes the different biological background of the CLL subgroups with mutated or unmutated *VH* and could in part explain their different clinical course. On the other hand, about two-thirds of the *VH*-unmutated CLL cases show no unfavorable genomic aberrations, indicating a differential influence of these factors (Table 1). In

Table 1 Relation of VH mutation status and genomic aberrations in 300 CLL cases (Kröber 2002)

Aberration	VH mutated (Homology <98%) n=132 (44%)	VH unmutated (Homology ≥98%) n=168 (56%)	p-Value *
Clonal aberrations	80%	84%	.37
13q deletion	65%	48%	.004
13q deletion single	50%	26%	<.001
Trisomy 12	15%	19%	.44
11q deletion	4%	27%	<.001
17p deletion	3%	10%	.03
17p or 11q deletion	7%	35%	<.001

* Fisher's exact test.

multivariate analysis the *VH* mutation status, 17p deletion, 11q deletion, age, leukocyte count, and LDH were identified as independent prognostic factors with regard to survival (Kröber 2002). The clinical stage of disease was not identified as an independent prognostic factor, indicating that in the knowledge of the genetic parameters the clinical stage of the disease may loose its independent prognostic value (Kröber 2002). Similar results, demonstrating a strong prognostic and independent impact of the *VH* mutation status and genomic aberrations, were found in two other series (Lin 2002; Oscier 2002). Therefore, four subgroups of CLL with markedly differing survival probabilities can be defined by the *VH* mutation status, 11q deletion, and 17p deletion (Fig. 3). Based on these studies it appears that *VH* mutation status and ge-

Fig. 2a,b Prognostic relevance of genomic aberrations in CLL (Döhner 2000). **a** Probabilities of disease progression as assessed by the treatment-free interval in the five dominant categories of genomic aberrations. The median treatment-free intervals for the 17p deletion (*n*=23), 11q deletion (*n*=56), 12q trisomy (*n*=47), normal karyotype (*n*=57), and 13q deletion (single abnormality; *n*=117) groups were 9, 13, 33, 49, and 92 months, respectively. **b** Estimated survival probabilities from the date of diagnosis in 325 CLL patients divided into the five categories defined in a hierarchical model of genomic aberrations in CLL (Döhner 2000). The median survival times for the 17p deletion (*n*=23), 11q deletion (*n*=56), 12q trisomy (*n*=47), normal karyotype (*n*=57), and 13q deletion (as single abnormality; *n*=117) groups were 32, 79, 114, 111, and 133 months, respectively

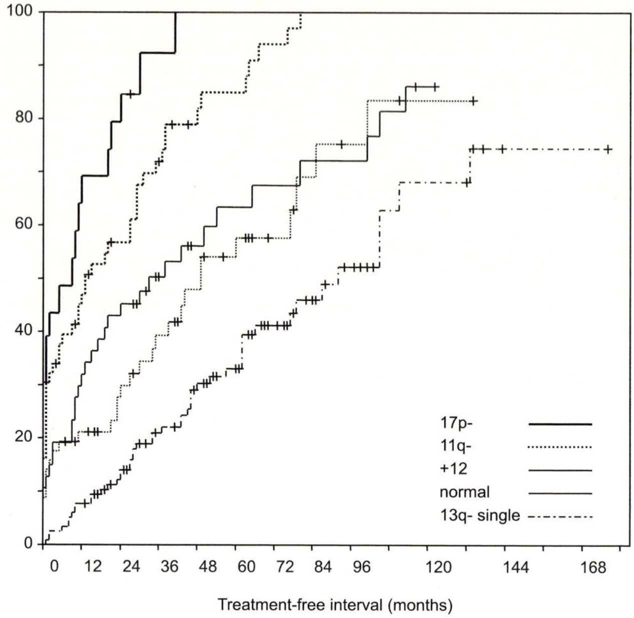
100
80
60
40
20
0
17p-
11q-
+12
normal
13q- single
0 12 24 36 48 60 72 84 96 120 144 168
Treatment-free interval (months)

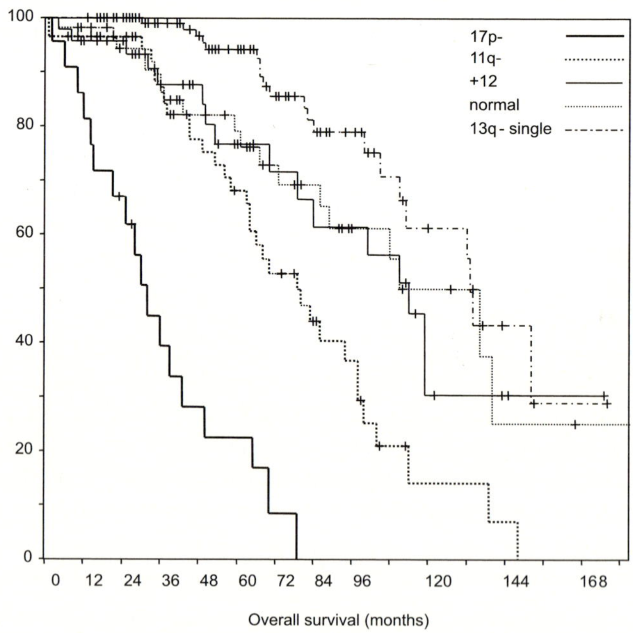
100
80
60
40
20
0
17p-
11q-
+12
normal
13q - single
0 12 24 36 48 60 72 84 96 120 144 168
Overall survival (months)

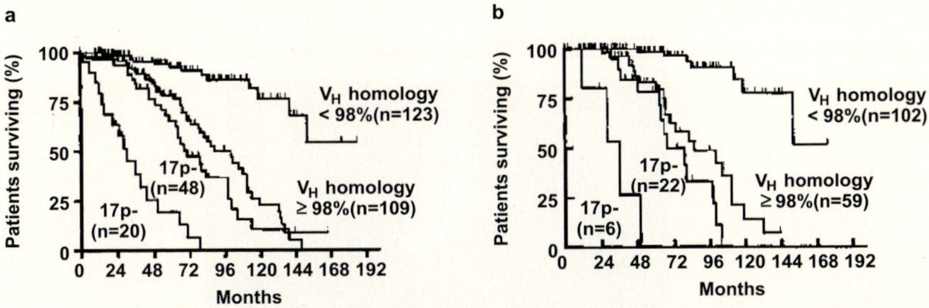

Fig. 3a, b Survival probabilities among patients in the following genetic categories: 17p⁻ (17p deletion irrespective of *VH* mutation status), 11q⁻ (11q deletion irrespective of *VH* mutation status), unmutated *VH* (homology≥98% and no 17p or 11q deletion), and mutated *VH* (homology<98% and no 17p or 11q deletion) (Kröber 2002). **a** Among all 300 patients estimated median survival times were: 17p⁻ 30m, 11q⁻ 70m, *VH*≥98% 89m, and *VH*<98% not reached (54% survival at 152m). **b** In Binet A patients only (n=189), estimated median survival times were: 17p⁻ 36m, 11q⁻ 68m, *VH*≥98% 86 months, and *VH*<98% not reached (52% survival at 152 months)

nomic aberrations are among the strongest currently available parameters and are of independent value to predict outcome in CLL.

2.3 Technical Developments and Future Diagnostic Tests

In order to further improve our understanding of the molecular pathomechanism and clinical outcome prediction, microarray platforms have been developed as tools to evaluate genome-wide parameters and defects. On the genomic level, matrix CGH (comparative genomic hybridization against a matrix of defined DNA fragments) is a sensitive test allowing the detection of novel recurrent aberrations of potential pathogenic and prognostic importance (Fig. 4) (Schwaenen 2004). On the gene expression level, comprehensive profiling studies of CLL based on DNA chip technology indicated that the global gene expression “signature” of *VH* mutated and unmutated CLL is very similar and that only the expression of a small number of genes discriminates between the two groups (Rosenwald 2001; Klein 2001). In addition to the characterization of expression signatures associated with the *VH* mutation subgroups of CLL, a study of 100 CLL samples characterized for the *VH* status and genomic aberrations described a significant number of differentially expressed genes clustering in chromosomal regions affected by the respective genomic losses or gains (Haslinger 2004). Deletions affecting chromosome bands 11q22–q23 and 17p13 led to a reduced expression of the genes in the corresponding genomic region, such as *ATM* and *p53*, while trisomy 12 resulted in

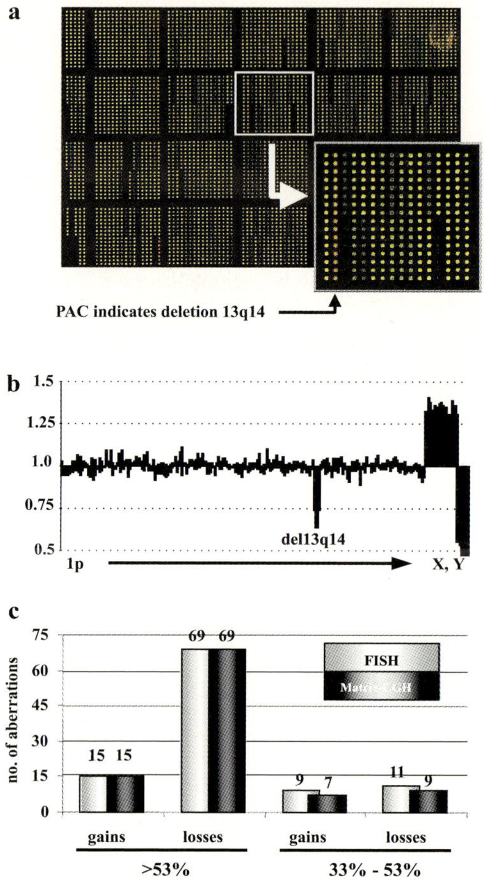

Fig. 4a–c Genome-wide diagnosis of genomic aberrations by matrix CGH (Schwänen 2004). **a** Image of a DNA chip after matrix CGH hybridization with DNA derived from a CLL patient carrying a 13q14 deletion (labeled in *green*; Cy3) versus human control DNA (labeled in *red*; Cy5). *Insert*: PAC clone in 13q14 with a dominantly red fluorescence signal after hybridization, indicating the deletion within this region (see *arrowhead*). **b** Example of a profile of signal ratios arranged in ascending chromosomal order beginning with 1p and ending with the X and Y chromosome. The cluster of fragments detecting deletion within 13q14 is indicated. In addition, the gender mismatch (CLL sample: female, control DNA sample: male) is detected by the imbalanced ratio of the X and Y chromosomes. **c** Assessment of the diagnostic power of the matrix CGH chip by comparison with data obtained by FISH with a comprehensive probe set. In 107 CLL displaying a total of 27 gains and 95 losses, all recurrently imbalanced regions were correctly identified, if the proportion of cells carrying the respective gains or losses was larger than 53% as determined by FISH

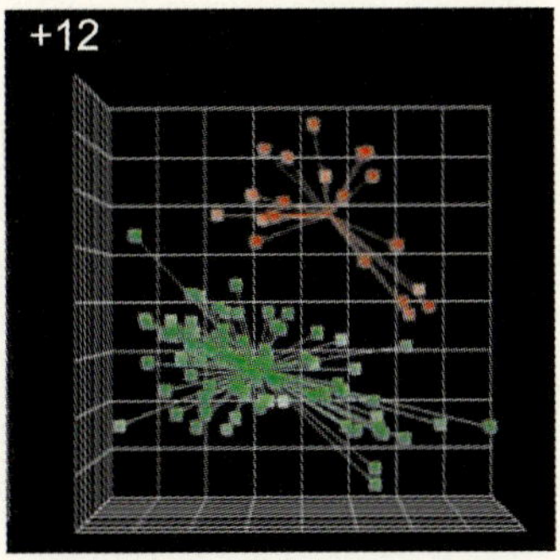

Fig. 5 Microarray gene expression analysis of CLL cases with or without trisomy 12 (Haslinger 2004). The principal component analysis of the first three principal components defined by the predictor variables shows a clear separation of the cases with trisomy 12 (*red symbols* in the *right upper quadrant*) from the cases without trisomy 12 (*green symbols* in the *lower left quadrant*) indicating distinct gene expression signatures when comparing CLL groups with different genomic aberrations

the upregulation of genes mapping to chromosome arm 12q (Fig. 5) (Kienle et al. 2005). The finding that the most significantly differentially expressed genes were located in the corresponding aberrant chromosomal regions indicates that a gene dosage effect may exert a pathogenic role in CLL.

3 Evaluation of Genotypic Factors in Clinical Trials

3.1 Progression in Early-Stage Disease

Distinct subgroups of CLL patients defined by specific genomic aberrations showed significantly different rates of disease progression in a retrospective series of heterogeneous patients (Fig. 2a). In addition, the prognostic impact of the *VH* mutation status and genomic aberrations with regard to overall survival was similarly observed for patients in early-stage disease (Binet A) as compared to advanced stage (Fig. 3).

In the prospective multicenter CLL1 trial of the German CLL Study Group (GCLLSG) CLL patients with Binet A disease are stratified into a high-risk arm if they have a lymphocyte doubling time (LDT) of less than 12 months and/or a diffuse bone marrow infiltration pattern, and a TK level greater than 7 U/l and/or β2-MG level greater than 3.5 mg/l (Bergmann 2003; see also http://www.dcllsg.de). Based on this stratification, the high-risk group is randomized between immediate treatment with fludarabine vs watch and wait, while the low-risk group is followed up. In addition, at enrollment genomic aberrations and *VH* mutation status are analyzed. These analyses show that high-risk aberrations ($11q^-$ or $17p^-$: 14%) and unmutated *VH* (41%) occur in a significant number of asymptomatic early-stage patients. When comparing the results from CLL1 with our single-center study containing patients diagnosed in all stages and the CLL4 study (Eichhorst 2003) [F vs FC (fludarabine vs fludarabine plus cyclophosphamide) for untreated Binet B/C patients, see also http://www.dcllsg.de], it is interesting to note that the incidence of low-risk markers (mutated *VH*, $13q^-$ single) is higher and the percentage of high-risk markers (unmutated *VH*, $11q^-$, $17p^-$) is lower. The low incidence of $11q^-$ in the CLL1 trial as compared to the other studies is likely due to the strong association of this abnormality with marked lymphadenopathy and rapid disease progression leading to recruitment of such patients in a trial for advanced-stage symptomatic disease.

In the CLL1 study, preliminary correlations of genetic parameters with progression-free survival (PFS) among untreated patients showed that unmutated *VH* as well as +12q, $11q^-$, and $17p^-$ are associated with more rapid disease progression (Stilgenbauer 2002a; Fig. 6). Moreover, the genetic parameters and the other parameters used for risk stratification appear to be correlated. Unmutated *VH* and high-risk aberrations ($17p^-$, $11q^-$, +12q) were significantly associated with the trial-defined high-risk group and with the individual parameters defining this group. However, there was discordance in 20%–40% of cases between individual parameters, i.e., among the trial-defined "high-risk" patients 37% had mutated *VH*, while in the "low-risk"

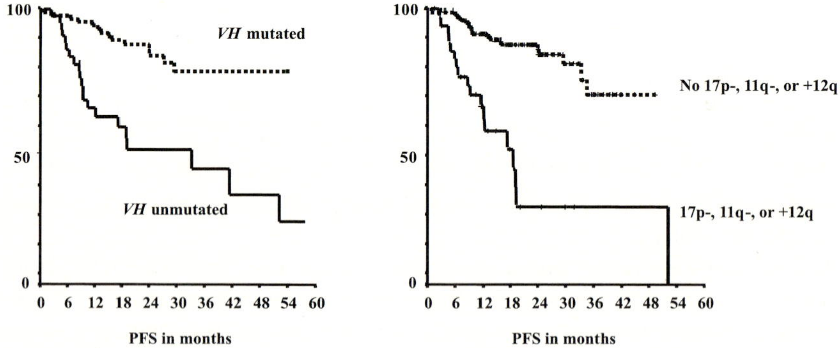

Fig. 6a, b Progression free survival (PFS) assessed according to genetic markers in the multicenter prospective CLL1 trial of the GCLLSG (Bergmann 2003; Stilgenbauer 2002a, see also http://www.dcllsg.de). **a** According to *VH* mutation status. **b** According to genomic aberrations group 28% had unmutated *VH*. In univariant analysis, the following prognostic indicators were significant for a shorter PFS: TK ($p<.001$), LDT ($p=.001$), lymphadenopathy ($p=.002$), β-MG ($p=.006$), absolute lymphocytes ($p=.004$), and unfavorable genomic aberrations ($11q^-$, $17p^-$, +12q) ($p<.001$), as well as unmutated *VH* status ($p=.003$). In multivariate analysis TK, LDT, and unfavorable genomic aberrations ($11q^-$, $17p^-$, +12q), as well as unmutated *VH* status were identified as independent variables. Therefore, it appears that a combination of several different factors may allow the best prediction of an individual patient's risk for disease progression. The upcoming CLL7 trial will therefore include the parameters TK, LDT, genomic aberrations, and *VH* mutation status for initial risk stratification among Binet A CLL patients. Furthermore, young early-stage patients in the "high-risk" group as defined in the CLL1 trial or by genetic risk factors (unmutated *VH*, $11q^-$, $17p^-$) and with active disease as defined by NCI criteria are eligible for the autologous and allogeneic transplantation protocols of the GCLLSG (see following section).

3.2
Response to Treatment in Advanced Disease

Genomic aberrations and *VH* mutation status influence the rate of disease progression, but with regard to overall survival additional parameters such as response to treatment are of importance. The fact that overall survival was inferior for the subgroups with unmutated *VH*, $11q^-$, or $17p^-$ despite the fact that comparable treatment modalities were used for patients with or without these markers indicates that response to therapy may be different in genetic subgroups (Döhner 2000; Kröber 2002).

In particular, the deletion $17p^-$ and/or abnormalities of the p53 gene involved in this aberration have been associated with failure after treatment with alkylating agents, purine analogs, and rituximab (El Rouby 1993; Geisler 1997; Döhner 1997; Byrd 2003). In a chromosome banding study of patients treated in a prospective trial based on alkylating agents, 17p aberrations were the only chromosomal aberration of prognostic relevance (Geisler 1997). An interphase-FISH study also showed that patients whose leukemia cells showed a $17p^-$/p53 deletion had significantly shorter survival times than patients without this aberration, and a relationship was found between the deletion and the response to treatment (Döhner 1995). While 56% of patients without the p53 deletion went into remission after treatment with purine-analogs, none of the patients with the p53 deletion showed a response. Similarly, the monoclonal anti-CD20 antibody rituximab did not show efficacy in CLL with the p53 deletion (Byrd 2003). In contrast, there is anecdotal evidence that durable therapeutic success can be achieved in CLL with the $17p^-$/p53 mutation using the monoclonal anti-CD52 antibody alemtuzumab (Stilgenbauer 2002b). This observation has been expanded in a retrospectively evaluated series of CLL cases mostly refractory to fludarabine therapy (Lozanski 2004). Treatment with intravenous alemtuzumab resulted in a complete remission (CR) or partial remission (PR) in 11 of 36 (31%) and in 6 of 15 (40%) patients with *p53* mutations or deletions. In the CLL2H study of the GCLLSG (alemtuzumab for fludarabine refractory CLL, see also http://www.dcllsg.de) a high incidence (27%) of $17p^-$ aberrations was observed, underlining the association of this abnormality with fludarabine-resistant disease. An interim analyses of this ongoing prospective trial has shown a response (CR or PR) in 10 of 21 *VH* unmutated, 5 of 10 $11q^-$, and 6 of 10 $17p^-$ cases, providing evidence from a controlled trial that alemtuzumab may be effective in CLL with the $17p^-$/*p53* mutation.

The observation that in a multivariate analysis $17p^-$, $11q^-$, and unmutated *VH* were independent adverse prognostic markers with regard to overall survival indicated that these factors may be associated with different outcomes after treatment. Validation of this concept is needed from prospective trials evaluating the best currently available prognostic markers in a controlled setting. *VH* mutation status, genomic aberrations, ZAP-70, etc. are currently being evaluated in different treatment trials from which, so far, only preliminary data have been available (Orchard 2003; Maloum 2003; Eichhorst 2003).

3.3 Risk Evaluation of Stem Cell Transplantation

Stem cell transplantation (SCT) is increasingly considered in the management of young patients with CLL, but these procedures may not only confer therapeutic benefit but are also associated with considerable toxicity and cost. The efficacy of autologous SCT relies solely on the cytotoxic therapy administered, while the anti-leukemic principle of allogeneic SCT adds the immune-mediated graft-vs-leukemia effect but also harbors the danger of graft-vs-host disease. There is a need to identify the role of prognostic factors which may be helpful to decide if a patient is a candidate for SCT or not and if an allogeneic SCT or autologous SCT should be considered. Whereas the first results of prospective trials (namely, the MRC pilot study and the GCLLSG CLL3 trial; see also http://www.dcllsg.de) confirm acceptable toxicity and effective but not durable disease control with *autologous* SCT in CLL (Dreger and Montserrat 2002; Milligan 2005), information on the influence of genetic risk factors on transplant outcome is limited. The transplant-related mortality (TRM) was 5% with a 2-year overall survival rate of 88% among 105 patients

(Dreger 2002). This result appears promising considering the high-risk features present in the majority of patients (CLL3 trial: 68% unmutated *VH*, 25% $11q^-$ or $17p^-$). However, the continuing occurrence of clinical and molecular relapse observed in all series on autologous SCT in CLL is evidence against the curative potential of the procedure in the majority of the patients.

Furthermore, genetic risk factors appear to retain their adverse impact after autologous SCT. The time to clinical relapse and the time to disease recurrence as assessed by CDR3 PCR was significantly shorter among patients with unmutated *VH* genes (Ritgen 2003). Nevertheless, the median treatment-free interval of 49 months in the *VH* unmutated cohort suggested a beneficial effect of autologous SCT for this high-risk population. This was confirmed in a matched-pair analysis of autologous SCT vs conventional treatment including the *VH* mutation status as matching variable (Dreger 2004). In this study, auto-SCT resulted in significantly longer overall survival as compared to conventional chemotherapy (autologous SCT: last death at 139 months, corresponding survival rate of 0.57, conventional: median survival 119 months) and this effect was primarily based on the benefit of the subgroup of cases with unmutated *VH* (Fig. 7).

As compared to autologous SCT, the primary therapeutic tool of allogeneic SCT after dose-reduced conditioning is the graft-vs-leukemia effect, which may offer long-term disease control and eventually a cure (Moreno et al. 2005; Sorror et al. 2005). Indeed, a recent comparative study of minimal residual disease (MRD) as detected by CDR3 PCR provided evidence that the graft-vs-leukemia effect is operational in CLL with unmutated *VH* (Ritgen 2004). In this study, only a modest decrease in MRD levels was observed immediately after

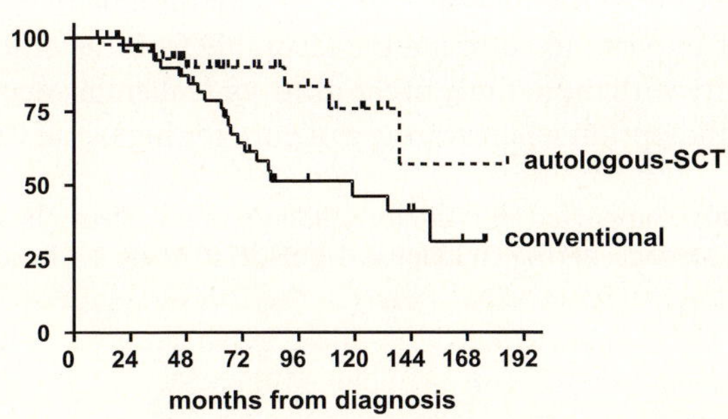

Fig. 7 Matched pair analysis based on the matching variables age, Binet stage, *VH* mutation status, and lymphocyte count between patients receiving autologous stem cell transplantation (autologous SCT) and conventional treatment (conventional; Dreger 2004). Survival from the time of diagnosis (n=88) of all patients treated with autologous SCT (*broken line*) and conventional chemotherapy (*solid line*)

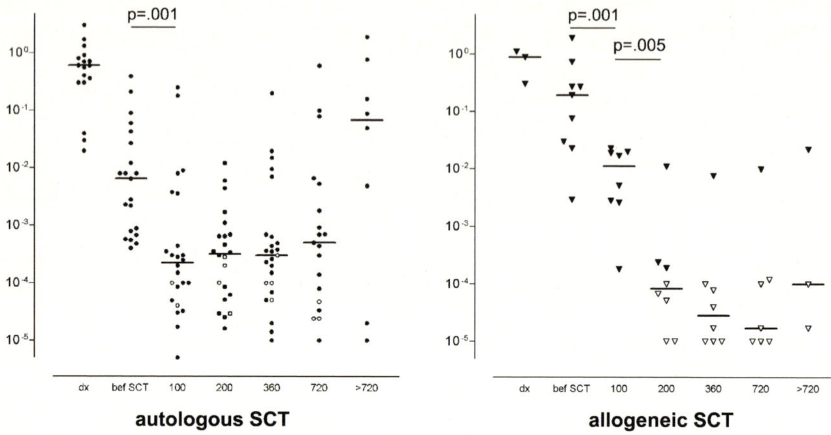

Fig. 8 MRD kinetics after autologous SCT and non-myeloablative allogeneic SCT (Ritgen 2004). MRD levels [number of CLL specific DNA copies per total DNA copies in the sample compared to the reference (pre-therapeutic) sample] of patients after myeloablative conditioning and auto-SCT and after non-myeloablative allogeneic SCT. *Black filled circles and triangles* denote MRD-positive samples whereas *blank circles and triangles* denote the sensitivity of PCR-negative samples (calculated minimum MRD level, which would have been detected in this particular sample)

allogeneic SCT, but MRD became undetectable in 7 of 9 (78%) CLL patients with unmutated *VH* after tapering immunosuppression, chronic graft-vs-host disease, or donor lymphocyte infusions. After a median of 25 (14–37) months, these 7 patients remain in clinical and molecular remission. In contrast, PCR negativity was achieved in only 6 of 26 (23%) control CLL cases with unmutated *VH* after autologous SCT and was not durable (Fig. 8). Therefore, allogeneic SCT appears to combine the favorable features of low treatment-related mortality with the activity of the graft-vs-leukemia effect, making this procedure a valid option when aiming at a cure for high-risk CLL.

Acknowledgements Supported by Wilhelm Sander-Stiftung, Deutsche Krebshilfe, Fresenius Stiftung, MedacSchering Onkologie GmbH, Hoffmann-La Roche AG and AMGEN GmbH.

References

Bergmann M, Eichhorst B, Busch R, Hallek M (2003) Elevated thymidine kinase and short lymphocyte doubling time in combination with unfavourable cytogenetics or unmutated IgVH status are strong predictors for high individual risk for rapid disease progression in patients with B-CLL in Binet stage A: an interim report from the CLL1 protocol of the German CLL Study Group (GCLLSG). Blood 102:Abstr 2464

Binet JL, Auquier A, Dighiero G, Chastang C, Piguet H, Goasguen J, Vaugier G, Potron G, Colona P, Oberling F, Thomas M, Tchernia G, Jaquillat C, Boivin P, Lesty C, Duaalt MT, Monconduit M, Belabbes S, Gremy F (1981) A new prognostic classification of chronic lymphocytic leukemia derived from a multivariate survival analysis. Cancer 48:198

Byrd JC, Smith L, Hackbarth ML, Flinn IW, Young D, Proffitt JH, Heerema NA (2003) Interphase cytogenetic abnormalities in chronic lymphocytic leukemia may predict response to rituximab. Cancer Res 63:36–38

Crespo M, Bosch F, Villamor N, Bellosillo B, Colomer D, Rozman M, Marce S, Lopez A, Campo E, Montserrat E (2003) ZAP-70 expression as a surrogate for immunoglobulin-variable-region mutations in chronic lymphocytic leukemia. N Engl J Med 348:1764–1775

Damle RN, Wasil T, Fais F, Ghiotto F, Valetto A, Allen SL, Buchbinder A, Budman D, Dittmar K, Kolitz J, Lichtman SM, Schulman P, Vinciguerra VP, Rai KR, Ferrarini M, Chiorazzi N (1999) Ig V gene mutation status and CD38 expression as novel prognostic indicators in chronic lymphocytic leukemia. Blood 94:1840

Dewald GW, Brockman SR, Paternoster SF, Bone ND, O'Fallon JR, Allmer C, James CD, Jelinek DF, Tschumper RC, Hanson CA, Pruthi RK, Witzig TE, Call TG, Kay NE (2003) Chromosome anomalies detected by interphase fluorescence in situ hybridization: correlation with significant biological features of B-cell chronic lymphocytic leukaemia. Br J Haematol 121:287–295

Di Giovanni S, Valentini G, Carducci P, Giallonardo P (1989) Beta-2-microglobulin is a reliable tumor marker in chronic lymphocytic leukemia. Acta Haematol 81:181

Dighiero G, Maloum K, Desablens B, Cazin B, Navarro M, Leblay R, Leporrier M, Jaubert J, Lepeu G, Dreyfus B, Binet JL, Tavade P, for the French Cooperative Groop on Chronic Lymphocytic Leukemia (1998) Chlorambucil in indolent chronic lymphocytic leukemia. N Engl J Med 21:1506

Döhner H, Fischer K, Bentz M, Hansen K, Benner A, Cabot G, Diehl D, Schlenk R, Coy J, Stilgenbauer S, Volkmann M, Galle PR, Poustka A, Hunstein W, Lichter P (1995) p53 gene deletion predicts for poor survival and non-response to therapy with purine analogs in chronic B-cell leukemias. Blood 85:1580–1589

Döhner H, Stilgenbauer S, Benner A, Leupolt E, Kröber A, Bullinger L, Döhner K, Bentz M, Lichter P (2000) Genomic aberrations and survival in chronic lymphocytic leukemia. N Engl J Med 343:1910–1916

Dreger P, Montserrat E (2002) Autologous and allogeneic stem cell transplantation for chronic lymphocytic leukemia. Leukemia 16:985–992

Dreger P, Stilgenbauer S, Benner A, Ritgen M, Kroeber A, Kneba M, Schmitz NDoehner H (2004) The prognostic impact of autologous stem cell transplantation in patients with chronic lymphocytic leukemia: a risk-matched analysis based on the VH gene mutational status. Blood 103:2850–2858

Eichhorst B, Busch R, Hopfinger G, Pasold R, Hensel M, Sölling U, Siehl S, Steinbrecher C, Jäger U, Bergmann M, Wendtner CM, Hiddemann W, Emmerich B, Hallek M (2003) Fludarabine plus cyclophosphamide (FC) induces higher remission rates and longer progression free survival (PFS) than fludarabine (F) alone in first line therapy of advanced chronic lymphocytic leukemia (CLL). Results of a phase III study (CLL4 protocol) of the German CLL Study Group (GCLLSG). Blood 102:Abstr 243

El Rouby S, Thomas A, Costin D, Rosenberg CR, Potmesil M, Silber R, Newcomb EW (1993) p53 gene mutation in B-cell chronic lymphocytic leukemia is associated with drug resistance and is independent of MDR1/MDR3 gene expression. Blood 82:3452–3459

Geisler CH, Philip P, Egelund Christensen B, Hou-Jensen K, Tinggaard Peterson N, Myhre Jensen O, Thorling K, Andersen E, Birgens HS, Drivsholm A, Ellegaard J, Larsen JK, Plesner T, Brown P, Kragh Andersen P, Mørk Hansen M (1997) In B-cell chronic lymphocytic leukaemia chromosome 17 abnormalities and not trisomy 12 are the single most important cytogenetic abnormalities for the prognosis: a cytogenetic and immunophenotypic study of 480 unselected newly diagnosed patients. Leuk Res 21:1011–1023

Ghia P, Guida G, Stella S, Gottardi D, Geuna M, Strola G, Scielzo C, Caligaris-Cappio F (2003) The pattern of CD38 expression defines a distinct subset of chronic lymphocytic leukemia (CLL) patients at risk of disease progression. Blood 101:1262–1269

Hallek M, Langenmayer I, Nerl C, Knauf W, Dietzfelbinger H, Adorf D, Ostwald M, Busch R, Kuhn-Hallek I, Thiel E, Emmerich B (1999) Elevated serum thymidine kinase levels identify a subgroup at high risk of disease progression in early, nonsmoldering chronic lymphocytic leukemia. Blood 93:1732

Hamblin TJ, Davis Z, Gardiner A, Oscier DG, Stevenson FK (1999) Unmutated Ig V(H) genes are associated with a more aggressive form of chronic lymphocytic leukemia. Blood 94:1848

Hamblin TJ, Orchard JA, Ibbotson RE, Davis Z, Thomas PW, Stevenson FK, Oscier DG (2002) CD38 expression and immunoglobulin variable region mutations are independent prognostic variables in chronic lymphocytic leukemia, but CD38 expression may vary during the course of the disease. Blood 99:1023–1029

Haslinger C, Schweifer N, Stilgenbauer S, Döhner H, Lichter P, Kraut N, Stratowa CAbseher R (2004) Microarray gene expression profiling of B-cell chronic lymphocytic leukemia subgroups defined by genomic aberrations and VH mutation status. J Clin Oncol 22:3937–3949

Kienle DL, Korz C, Hosch B, Benner A, Mertens D, Habermann A, Kröber A, Jäger U, Lichter P, Döhner H, Stilgenbauer S (2005) Evidence for distinct pathomechanisms in genetic subgroups of chronic lymphocytic leukemia revealed by quantitative expression analysis of cell cycle, activation, and apoptosis associated genes. J Clin Oncol (Epub ahead of print)

Klein U, Tu Y, Stolovitzky GA, Mattioli M, Cattoretti G, Husson H, Freedman A, Inghirami G, Cro L, Baldini L, Neri A, Califano A, Dalla-Favera R (2001) Gene expression profiling of B cell chronic lymphocytic leukemia reveals a homogeneous phenotype related to memory B cells. J Exp Med 194:1625–1638

Kröber A, Seiler T, Benner A, Bullinger L, Brückle E, Lichter P, Döhner H, Stilgenbauer S (2002) VH mutation status, CD38 expression level, genomic aberrations, and survival in chronic lymphocytic leukemia. Blood 100:1410–1416

Lin K, Sherrington PD, Dennis M, Matrai Z, Cawley JC, Pettitt AR (2002) Relationship between p53 dysfunction, CD38 expression, and IgV(H) mutation in chronic lymphocytic leukemia. Blood 100:1404–1409

Lozanski G, Heerema NA, Flinn IW, Smith L, Harbison J, Webb J, Moran M, Lucas M, Lin T, Hackbarth ML, Proffitt JH, Lucas D, Grever MR, Byrd JC (2004) Alemtuzumab is an effective therapy for chronic lymphocytic leukemia with p53 mutations and deletions. Blood 103:3278–3281

Maloum K, Magnac C, Cazin B, Divine M, Lepretre S, Delmer A, Leporrier M, Jaubert J, Dreyfus B, Guibon O, Dighiero G, Merle-Beral H (2003) Expression of unmutated VH genes is a detrimental prognostic factor in chronic lymphocytic leukemia predictive value of mutational IgVH gene status for incomplete response and relapse after oral fludarabine phosphate (Fludara oral) and cyclophosphamide in previously untreated CLL patients. Blood 102:Abstr 110

Milligan DW, Fernandes S, Dasgupta R, Davies FE, Matutes E, Fegan CD, McConkey C, Child JA, Cunningham D, Morgan GJ, Catovsky D; National Cancer Research Institute Haematological Studies Group (2005) Results of the MRC pilot study show autografting for younger patients with chronic lymphocytic leukemia is safe and achieves a high percentage of molecular responses. Blood 105:397–404

Moreno C, Villamor N, Colomer D, Esteve J, Martino R, Nomdedu J, Bosch F, Lopez-Guillermo A, Campo E, Sierra J, Montserrat E (2005) Allogeneic stem-cell transplantation may overcome the adverse prognosis of unmutated VH gene in patients with chronic lymphocytic leukemia. J Oncol (Epub ahead of print)

Montserrat E, Sanchez-Bisono J, Vinolas N, Rozman C (1986) Lymphocyte doubling time in chronic lymphocytic leukaemia: analysis of its prognostic significance. Br J Haematol 62:567

Orchard J, Davis Z, Ibbotson R, Richards S, Catovsky D, Oscier D (2003) Comparison of ZAP-70, IgVHgene mutational status and CD38 in CLL patients requiring therapy: preliminary report from the UK CLL IV Trial. Blood 102:Abstr 105

Oscier DG, Gardiner AC, Mould SJ, Glide S, Davis ZA, Ibbotson RE, Corcoran MM, Chapman RM, Thomas PW, Copplestone JA, Orchard JA, Hamblin TJ (2002) Multivariate analysis of prognostic factors in CLL: clinical stage, IGVH gene mutational status, and loss or mutation of the p53 gene are independent prognostic factors. Blood 100:1177–1184

Rai KR, Sawitsky A, Cronkite EP, Chanana AD, Levy RN, Paternack BS (1975) Clinical staging of chronic lymphocytic leukemia. Blood 46:219

Ritgen M, Lange A, Stilgenbauer S, Dohner H, Bretscher C, Bosse H, Stuhr A, Kneba M, Dreger P (2003) Unmutated immunoglobulin variable heavy chain gene status remains an adverse prognostic factor after autologous stem cell transplantation for chronic lymphocytic leukemia. Blood 101:2049–2053

Ritgen M, Stilgenbauer S, von Neuhoff N, Humpe A, Bruggemann M, Pott C, Raff T, Kröber A, Bunjes D, Schlenk R, Schmitz N, Döhner H, Kneba M, Dreger P (2004) Graft-versus-leukemia activity may overcome therapeutic resistance of chronic lymphocytic leukemia with unmutated immunoglobulin variable heavy chain gene status: implications of minimal residual disease measurement with quantitative PCR. Blood 104:2600–2602

Rosenwald A, Alizadeh AA, Widhopf G, Simon R, Davis RE, Yu X, Yang L, Pickeral OK, Rassenti LZ, Powell J, Botstein D, Byrd JC, Grever MR, Cheson BD, Chiorazzi N, Wilson WH, Kipps TJ, Brown PO, Staudt LM (2001) Relation of gene expression phenotype to immunoglobulin mutation genotype in B cell chronic lymphocytic leukemia. J Exp Med 194:1639–1647

Rozman C, Montserrat E, Rodriguez-Fernandez JM, Ayats R, Vallespi T, Parody R, Rios A, Prados D, Morey M, Gomis F, Alcala A, Gutierrez M, Maldonado J, Gonzales C, Giralt M, Hernandez-Nieto L, Cabrera A, Fernandez-Ranada JM (1984) Bone marrow histologic pattern—the best single prognostic parameter in chronic lymphocytic leukemia: a multivariate survival analysis of 329 cases. Blood 64:642

Schwaenen C, Nessling M, Wessendorf S, Salvi T, Wrobel G, Radlwimmer B, Kestler HA, Haslinger C, Stilgenbauer S, Dohner H, Bentz M, Lichter P (2004) Automated array-based genomic profiling in chronic lymphocytic leukemia: development of a clinical tool and discovery of recurrent genomic alterations. Proc Natl Acad Sci U S A 101:1039–1044

Stilgenbauer S, Döhner H (2002b) Campath-1H induced complete remission of chronic lymphocytic leukemia despite p53 gene mutation and resistance to chemotherapy. N Engl J Med 347:452–453 (letter)

Stilgenbauer S, Kröber A, Winkler D, Kienle D, Busch R, Emmerich B, Hallek M, Döhner H, for the GCLLSG (2002a) VH mutation status and genomic aberrations in the prospective CLL1 trial (Binet-A) of the German CLL Study Group (GCLLSG). Blood 100:168a (Abstr 628)

Sorror ML, Maris MB, Sandmaier BM, Storer BE, Stuart MJ, Hegenbart U, Agura E, Chauncey TR, Leis J, Pulsipher M, McSweeney P, Radich JP, Bredeson C, Bruno B, Langston A, Loken MR, Al-Ali H, Blume KG, Storb R, Maloney DG (2005) Hematopoietic cell transplantation after nonmyeloablative conditioning for advanced chronic lymphocytic leukemia. J Clin Oncol (Epub ahead of print)

Tobin G, Thunberg U, Johnson A, Thorn I, Soderberg O, Hultdin M, Botling J, Enblad G, Sallstrom J, Sundstrom C, Roos G, Rosenquist R (2002) Somatically mutated Ig V(H)3-21 genes characterize a new subset of chronic lymphocytic leukemia. Blood 99:2262–2264

Vasconcelos Y, Davi F, Levy V, Oppezzo P, Magnac C, Michel A, Yamamoto M, Pritsch O, Merle-Beral H, Maloum K, Ajchenbaum-Cymbalista F, Dighiero G (2003) Binet's staging system and VH genes are independent but complementary prognostic indicators in chronic lymphocytic leukemia. J Clin Oncol 21:3928–3932

Zwiebel JA, Cheson BD (1998) Chronic lymphocytic leukemia: staging and prognostic factors. Semin Oncol 25:42

CTMI (2005) 294:165–185

Chronic Lymphocytic Leukaemia: Clinical Translations of Biological Features

T. J. Hamblin (✉)

Department of Haematology, Royal Bournemouth Hospital, Castle Lane East, Bournemouth BH7 7DW, UK
terjoha@aol.com

Abstract The chronic lymphatic leukaemia (CLL) world was surprised to find that the disease split so neatly down the middle into those patients with unmutated immunoglobulin genes who were mainly men, had aggressive disease and were destined to die from their disease, on average at about 8 years from diagnosis, and those with mutated immunoglobulin genes who were equally distributed between the sexes, had indolent disease and usually died of something else a quarter of a century later. This discovery gave fresh impetus to the investigation into the biology of CLL. We now know more about, though we are still not certain of, the cell of origin of the disease and how it functions and fails to function. Intriguing clues about the roles of infectious agents and the functioning of the immune response have been scattered, but not quite put together. In addition, clinicians have been given a new tool for determining prognosis, though the tool is too clumsy for day-to-day use and surrogates are being sought. Treatment strategies based on the new biology are in development.

1 The Heterogeneous Nature of Chronic Lymphocytic Leukaemia

We have always known that chronic lymphocytic leukaemia (CLL) was a very heterogeneous disease. Some patients die within 2 years of diagnosis, others live to a great age with scarcely a movement in their white count—it remains at the same slightly raised level that drew attention to the diagnosis 35 years previously. So unpredictable has been the prognosis that the standard management of early-stage CLL has been to delay treatment until something happens (CLL Trialists' Collaborative Group 1999). This seems equivalent to a tennis player watching to see which way the ball will bounce before deciding on the shot to play, but on the basis of knowledge available in 1999 there was firm evidence that this was the best policy. For the patient the situation was unsatisfactory. The doctor called it 'watch and wait', the patient called it 'watch and worry'. To change the sporting metaphor, we needed to be able to tell Shane Warne's leg break from his googly before the ball bounced.

At first, CLL experts suspected that the heterogeneity was caused by the contamination of the diagnosis by CLL look-alikes. Immunophenotyping unravelled that. Even when cases of mantle cell lymphoma, splenic lymphoma with villous lymphocytes and various other spillover lymphomas were eliminated the heterogeneity remained. Yet CLL seemed a very 'pure' disease. Granted, there is no karyotypic unity, but the immunophenotype is unique: CD5 positive, CD23 positive, CD79b weak or negative, FMC7 negative and surface immunoglobulin (Ig) weak (Moreau et al. 1997). It seems unlikely that any other B cell tumour would resemble that.

The CD5 positivity and other similarities seemed to point to an origin of the tumour from follicular mantle cells, and hence from cells yet to enter the germinal centre (Caligaris-Cappio 1996). It was, therefore, to be expected that CLL cells would have Ig variable region (*IgV*) genes that had not been subjected to somatic mutation, a process believed to occur only in the germinal centre (Jacob et al. 1991; Berek et al. 1991). Sure enough, early papers confirmed this expectation (Kipps et al. 1989; Deane and Norton 1991; Ebeling et al. 1992). There were, however, sufficient exceptions to worry those with an open mind. The review by Schroeder and Dighiero (1994) startled the cognoscenti by revealing that only half the published cases had unmutated *IgV* genes while those of the other half were mutated. Closer scrutiny of the published cases uncovered a few CLL impostors that were CD5 negative, but the majority of those with mutated genes were true-blue CLL.

This review was instrumental in undoing one of the givens of CLL and was a spur to further studies. Was it conceivable that CLL was two diseases? One line of investigation was to study the karyotype. Perhaps the various chromosomal abnormalities in CLL were late changes that induced secondary variation on the basic pattern. An early, and often neglected, paper demonstrated that trisomy 12, then thought to be the commonest abnormality in CLL, was usually associated with unmutated *IgV* genes, while deletion at 13q14 (actually the commonest abnormality) was usually associated with mutated *IgV* genes (Oscier et al. 1997). Since CLL with trisomy 12 has a worse prognosis than CLL with deletions at 13q14 we decided to look at a larger series and examine prognosis. Astonishingly, there was a huge difference in survival in patients with differing patterns of mutations. Those with unmutated *IgV* genes had a median survival of about 8 years, while those with mutated *IgV* genes had a median survival of nearly 25 years (Hamblin et al. 1999). Quite independently, colleagues in New York and Italy found identical outcomes and both papers were published alongside each other in the same issue of *Blood* (Damle et al. 1999; Hamblin et al. 1999). Several other groups have since confirmed the findings, and this is now the new paradigm (Maloum et al. 2000; Bahler et al. 2000; Jelinek et al. 2001; Krober et al. 2002; Lin et al. 2002).

The suggestion was made that CLL is really two diseases, one arising from naïve B cells that have yet to meet antigen and one arising from memory B cells that have encountered antigen and in response have undergone somatic mutation in the germinal centre (Hamblin et al. 2002).

2
How Significantly Do the Two Types of CLL Differ from Each Other?

Traditionally, CLL has been thought of as a disease with a male preponderance. Strictly speaking this is only true for cases with unmutated *IgV* genes (which for convenience I shall call U-CLL), where the gender ratio is about 3:1. In contrast, for those with mutated *IgV* genes (M-CLL) the ratio between the sexes is close to unity (Fig. 1). In some ways the difference in the gender ratio is the strongest evidence that we are dealing with two diseases.

Although there is great similarity between the morphology of all cases of CLL, haematopathologists recognize atypical pictures either with excess prolymphocytes or with an admixture of cells with cleaved nuclei and lymphoplasmacytoid cells (Bennett et al. 1989; Matutes et al. 1996). Atypical morphology is significantly more common in U-CLL than M-CLL (Hamblin et al. 1999).

Survival curves for the two subsets continue to show a marked difference even though the series of cases has been greatly expanded. This difference is emphasized by removing from analysis deaths from unrelated causes,

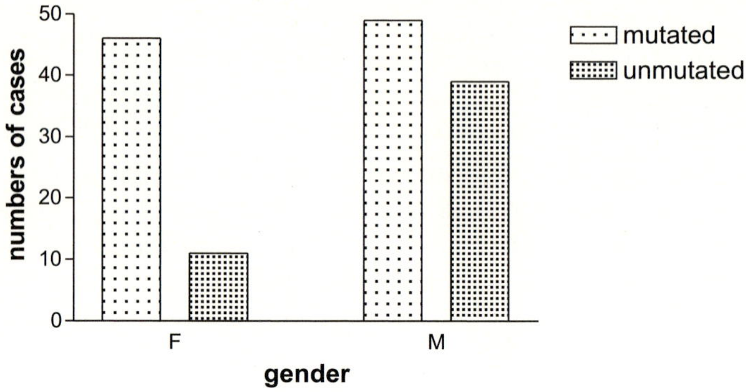

Fig. 1 Gender ratio of cases of CLL with mutated and unmutated *IgV* genes (145 cases)

though this is difficult to assess in multi-centre studies. However, since the Bournemouth series comprises mainly local cases we have been able to do this with some assurance (Fig. 2). In general, patients with M-CLL do not die from their CLL whereas patients with U-CLL almost invariably do, should they avoid a very early death from heart disease, stroke or other malignancy.

M-CLL is a disease in which the lymphocyte count is stable or only slowly increasing. In contrast, U-CLL is usually associated with progressive disease (Fig. 3). In a few patients U-CLL has a biphasic course, a period of stability being followed by acceleration. This may coincide with an added genetic change such as the acquisition of *p53* mutations or deletion of one copy of

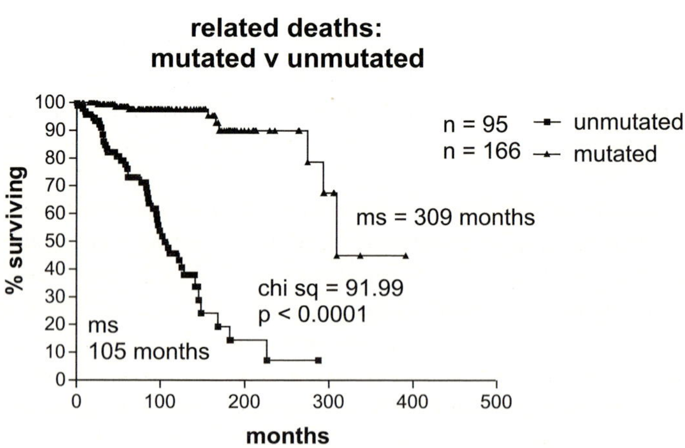

Fig. 2 Survival curve M-CLL versus U-CLL, censored for deaths unrelated to CLL (n=261). *PROG*, progressive

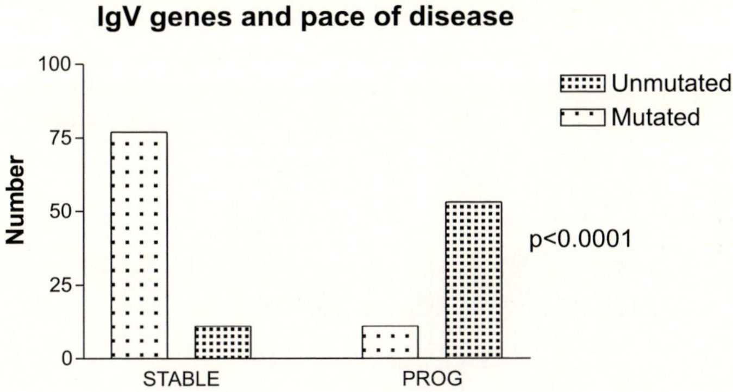

Fig. 3 Comparison of pace of disease in M-CLL and U-CLL (145 cases)

ATM on chromosome 11q23, (Oscier et al. 2002; Lin et al. 2002; Krober et al. 2002) but in individual cases that evidence is often lacking. Although genetic progression of this sort may occur in M-CLL (where its malign significance has yet to be established), it is much more likely in U-CLL.

This is not to say that M-CLL is entirely benign. In many cases the lymphocyte count continues to rise, though rarely having a doubling time of less than 12 months. Lymph nodes and spleen enlarge, though rarely massively. Richter's syndrome can occur occasionally. Late in the disease (after having it for 20 years), hypogammaglobulinaemia is often seen. The other major complication of CLL, autoimmune haemolytic anaemia, does occur in M-CLL. In our series, the overall incidence is 11.4%; in M-CLL it is 7.2% and in U-CLL it is 18.2%.

The idea that the disease is more severe in young people seems to be a myth. In our series the ratio between M-CLL and U-CLL is the same at every age of presentation, except in the very elderly, where U-CLL predominates, probably because physicians are less likely to inflict unnecessary blood tests on well old people (Fig. 4).

Nowadays, most patients present with early-stage disease. In our hands, 76% present because of an incidental blood test. The majority of patients who present with Binet stage B or C disease have U-CLL (Fig. 5). Some patients with M-CLL present with advanced disease. The problem with these is in knowing how long the patient has had CLL. It is clinically silent until the patient has a blood test, and these are not compulsory even in countries with socialized medicine. The true prevalence of CLL is not known, though a monoclonal population of lymphocytes with the immunophenotype of CLL cells may be found in the blood of 3.5% of the population over 40 years of age (Rawstron et al. 2002).

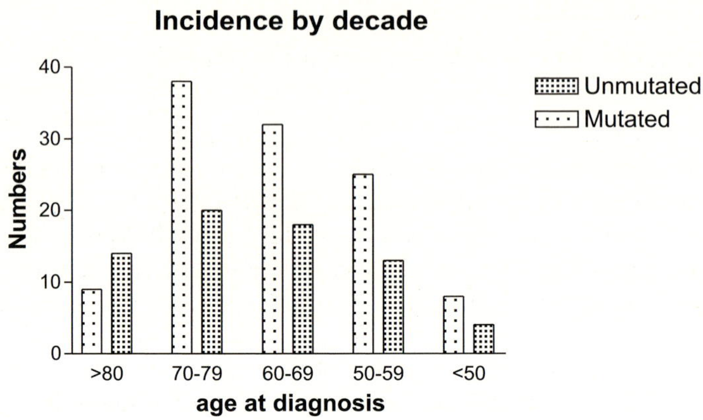

Fig. 4 Incidence of M-CLL and U-CLL with age (145 cases)

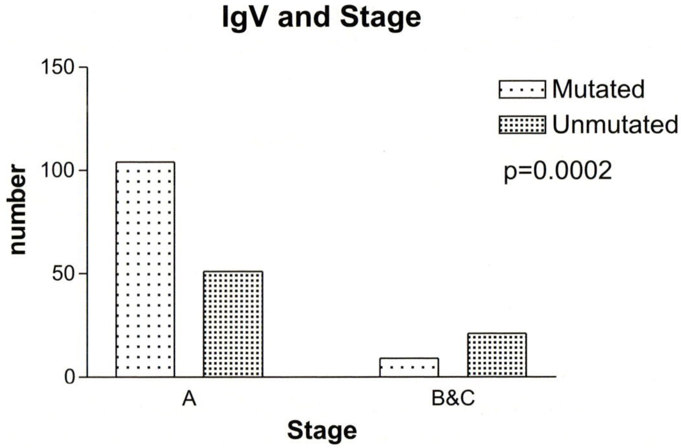

Fig. 5 Comparison of presenting Binet stage in M-CLL and U-CLL (178 cases)

Although stage is an important prognostic factor, mutational status is more so. In our hands, advanced-stage M-CLL patients live for twice as long as advanced stage U-CLL patients, and early-stage U-CLL patients survive for only a year longer than advanced stage U-CLL patients (manuscript in preparation). When treatment becomes necessary in M-CLL, patients survive about twice as long as patients with U-CLL after their first treatment (manuscript in preparation). Similarly, relapse after stem cell autograft is significantly delayed in M-CLL compared to U-CLL (Ritgen et al. 2003).

From a clinical point of view, these look like two separate diseases, heavily disguised to look like each other.

3
Challenging the New Paradigm: Not Two But One

As ever, technology drives science. Two papers, again appearing alongside each other—this time in the *Journal of Experimental Medicine*—reported on the new technique of gene expression profiling as applied to CLL (Klein et al. 2001; Rosenwald et al. 2001). Despite using different techniques, both papers had the same message: CLL has a distinct genetic signature that distinguishes it from other lymphomas and normal B lymphocytes. The genes expressed by the two subsets were remarkably similar. One paper found that the difference between the two was in the expression of fewer than 30 genes among more than 12,000. The other found that around 175 genes were differently expressed in the two subsets out of over 17,000 studied.

Klein et al. (2001) also demonstrated that the genes expressed in CLL cells more closely resembled those of naïve and memory cells than those of either germinal centre B cells or normal CD5-positive B cells, and although there were some discrepancies, both subsets were closer to the pattern of memory cells than naïve cells. We were thus confronted with the possibility that CLL is a tumour of memory B cells existing in two subtypes, but essentially one disease.

4
CLL: A Tumour of Memory B Cells?

Memory cells are so called because they 'remember' an encounter with antigen and have been altered so as to respond to the next encounter in an enhanced way. This idea is easy to accept for cells with hypermutated *IgV* genes, and indeed there is good evidence that the somatic mutations in M-CLL have occurred according to the standard germinal centre process (Messmer et al. 2003). The antigenic encounter has triggered a series of reactions that produce an altered B cell receptor (BCR) that fits more snugly with the antigen and enables the cell to respond more efficiently in future.

According to the textbook model (MacLennan 1994), the generation of memory cells requires the formation of a germinal centre. The germinal centre is the morphological arrangement that facilitates this process, being initiated when antigen-presenting cells (such as interdigitating dendritic cells) present antigens to CD4-positive T cells in the T cell zones of peripheral lymph organs. In the meantime, follicular B cells, as a consequence of their BCR-engaging antigen, migrate into T cell areas and undergo cognate co-stimulatory interactions with these T cells. These interactions trigger changes in the B cells, which then migrate back into the follicle where, in the context of the stromal environment provided by follicular dendritic cells, they rapidly divide. The rapidly dividing B cells are blast-like (centroblasts), express little surface Ig and occupy the dark zone of the emerging germinal centre. It is here that the generation of mutant clones occurs. The light zone is occupied by secondary follicular dendritic cells and CD4-positive T cells. It is to this zone that the B cells next migrate changing as they do into centrocytes and expressing greater quantities of Ig on their surface. The light zone can be seen as the test bed where the affinity of the mutant BCR for antigen is assessed. Cells reacting poorly are destined for apoptosis.

The precise mechanism by which somatic hypermutation is produced is unclear, but the induction of activation-induced cytidine deaminase (AID) is a necessary prerequisite (Muramatsu et al. 2000). The other function of the germinal centre, isotype switching, is also under the control of this enzyme. Thus, both somatic hypermutation and Ig class switching act as a sort of visa stamp that a cell has passed through the germinal centre.

5
How Can a Cell with Unmutated *IgV* Genes Be Thought of as a Memory Cell?

Whether the *IgV* genes are mutated or unmutated, there are certainly signs that the CLL cell has been stimulated by something. The upregulation of CD23, CD25, CD69, CD71 and even CD5 is evidence of activation, as is the downregulation of CD22, CD79b, FcγIIb and IgD (Chiorazzi and Ferrarini 2003). All CLL cells express CD27, often thought to be a marker of memory B cells (van Oers et al. 1993; Lens et al. 1996).

There are also signs that both subsets have encountered antigen. The use of the 51 *IgV* heavy chain genes by CLL is not random. The most commonly used gene is *V1-69*, predominantly the 51p1 polymorphism (Fais et al. 1997; Johnson et al. 1997; Hamblin et al. 1999). This is not merely an age effect. The elderly use *V1-69* no more commonly than younger people in their normal repertoire (Potter et al. 2003; Brezinschek et al. 1998). The overuse of *V1-69* is mainly in the unmutated subset and it is usually found in association with the *D3-3* gene segment in the second reading frame and *JH6* (Johnson et al. 1997). This results in a very long complementarity determining region 3 (CDR3) that is tyrosine rich and very acidic (Chiorazzi and Ferrarini 2003).

An even more remarkable biased association has been reported by Chiorazzi and Ferrarini (2003). They report five cases of CLL all expressing unmutated surface IgG. They all used *V4-39*, *D6-13* and *JH5* for the heavy chain and for the light chain the same unmutated *O12/2* gene together with *Jκ1*, leading to a virtually identical antibody combining site in all cases.

A similar preferential pairing has been found for the *V3-21* gene. This group of cases almost always uses the *JH6* gene and has a very short CDR3 caused by deletions of D segment nucleotides. They also tend to use the $V_\lambda 2\text{-}14/J_\lambda 3$ light chain genes (Tobin et al. 2003). This interesting group of patients stands out by having an equally bad prognosis whether the genes are mutated or unmutated (Tobin et al. 2002). Although this finding was originally thought to be local to the Baltic region, latest results from the British CLL4 trial have identified the same phenomenon there (D.G. Oscier, personal communication).

Other less-emphatic associations have been reported such as both *V3-07* and *V4-34* preferentially associated with *JH4* with a short CDR3 in the mutated subset (Chiorazzi and Ferrarini 2003). Scrutiny of a larger database may uncover others. The most likely explanation for all these biases is the selection by antigen of particular conformations of the BCR. The nature of the antigen is unclear. It could be a common pathogen, though as yet none has been suggested. However, we live in an age when new infectious agents are readily and unexpectedly discovered to be the cause of old diseases. It could be autoantigen. The surface Ig of CLL cells has long been known to react with self-antigens in a multispecific, low-affinity manner (Broker et al. 1988).

If all CLL cells have encountered antigen, how then does the unmutated subset remain unmutated? It is possible that passage through the germinal centre requires no alteration of the BCR since it already reacts well with the putative antigen. If this were the case it is difficult to see why this should confer a uniformly worse prognosis. Alternatively, the BCR might be stimulated outside the context of the germinal centre. Chiorazzi and Ferrarini (2001) have suggested that the cells have responded to T-independent antigens. Stevenson and Caligaris-Cappio (2004) have suggested that they might be responding to superantigen. A superantigen is one that binds to framework regions of the Ig variable regions. Such 'antigens' are known to be able to cause the expansion of B cells (Silverman 1997). Neither explanation is wholly satisfactory. As we shall see, the proliferation of U-CLL cells occurs in a sea of T cells, and the *IgV* biases include the whole CDR-3, not just the framework regions.

The situation is complicated by the fact that the U-CLL subset includes patients with small numbers of mutations. Originally a 2% divergence from the germline was allowed because of an unknown number of polymorphisms that might account for slight changes. However, by comparing *IgV* sequences in CLL cells and neutrophils from the same patients, Davis et al. (2003) were able to show that even these few variations were true mutations. Given that that is true, the question arises as to exactly how many mutations can be

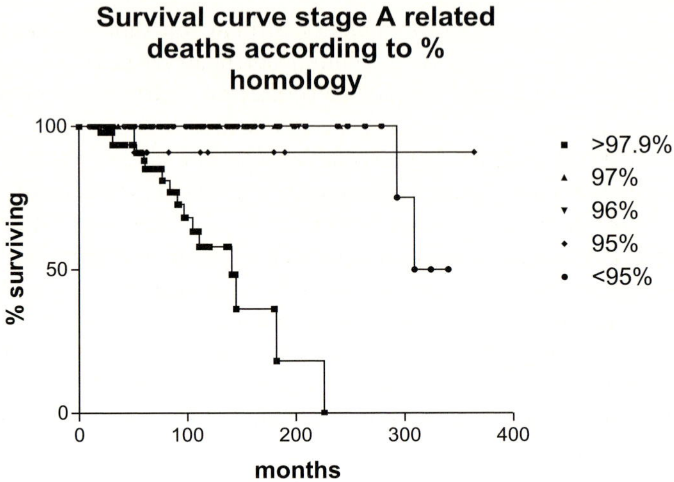

Fig. 6 Survival curve showing survival of patients with Binet stage A CLL comparing those with >97.9% *IgV* gene sequence homology to the germline with those with 97%–97.9%, 96%–96.9%, 95%–95.9% and <95% homology, censored for deaths unrelated to CLL. There was only one early death in a patient with <98% sequence homology, and she had <96% sequence homology (*n*=145)

allowed until a case falls outside the U-CLL subgroup. Suggestions have been made that greater than 97% homology or even greater than 95% homology might be a better cut-off (Krober et al. 2002; Lin et al. 2002). However, in our hands, Youden's index indicated that greater than 98% gave the sharpest separation (Hamblin et al. 1999). A reanalysis with greater numbers of cases confirms this view, especially when it is confined to Binet stage A patients (since we do not have a start date for advanced-stage patients) and deaths unrelated to CLL are censored (Fig. 6).

In an individual case of CLL, the mutational signature has been thought to be close to constant in all the cells. This differs from the story in follicular lymphoma where a family tree exposing the mutational history can be constructed from the various sub-clones (Zhu et al. 1994). The cell is thought to be trapped in the microenvironment of the germinal centre, perhaps caused by the acquisition of potential N-glycosylation sites in the *IgV* region by somatic mutation (Zhu et al. 2002). However, it is now clear that somatic mutation may occur outside the germinal centre (Weller et al. 2001; Toellner et al. 2002), though at a lesser rate than within the germinal centre. Unexpectedly, it seems that the mutational signature in CLL is not stable, but perhaps in the majority of cases (Gurrieri et al. 2002) new mutations continue to be generated and occasionally subclones emerge.

This may be related to the detection of AID in CLL cells (McCarthy et al. 2003; Albesiano et al. 2003; Oppezzo et al. 2003), which seems to preferentially occur in U-CLL, though one paper suggests that its occurrence is in only a tiny fraction of the cells.

Hence, confusion reigns. The malignant cell in U-CLL gives the appearance of having encountered antigen but in an unconventional way. The mutational process seems functional, but if begun at all has been abruptly aborted. Mutation of the *IgV* genes may occur outside a germinal centre, but whether this has occurred in a minimal way in U-CLL is unclear.

Thus, 'memory cell' is probably an unsuitable name. I prefer the concept of an 'antigen experienced' cell, implying that here is a cell that has experienced contact with antigen, has changed somewhat so that it is 'ready' for another experience, but has not changed sufficiently by mutating its *IgV* genes to have learnt from its experience.

6 Stimulation Outside the Context of the Germinal Centre

The availability of tumour cells at the end of a needle has made CLL the easiest tumour to investigate, but these cells are peripheral to the proliferative process. Proliferation takes place in proliferation centres, sometimes known as pseudofollicles. These are nodular areas in lymph nodes and bone marrow that lack mantles. They comprise aggregates of prolymphocytes together with CD4-positive T cells many of which express CD40 ligand. There is dispute as to whether pseudofollicles contain follicular dendritic cells (Moreton et al. 2003; Schmid and Isaacson 1994). They differ from reactive follicles in not expressing Bcl-6 and CD10, and in being Bcl-2 positive (Schmid and Isaacson 1994). The CLL cells in the pseudofollicle have a unique phenotype, being Mum-1 positive, Ki-67 positive, Oct-2 positive, Bob-1 positive and CD71 positive (Moreton et al. 2003).

Although both M-CLL and U-CLL have proliferation centres, Bahler et al. (2000) found that they were in different relationships to reactive follicles in the two subsets. Elison et al. (1989) had previously described two types of small lymphocytic lymphoma (the nodal equivalent of CLL) in one of which proliferation centres were encamped around reactive follicles, while in the other the proliferation centres were localized between reactive follicles. Bahler et al. found that the former type tended to have mutated *IgV* genes and the latter unmutated. If this work can be confirmed it is further evidence that CLL comprises one process applied to two different types of cell. Such a concept is compatible with the microarray picture, since the 'one process' involves the upregulation and downregulation of one set of genes, and compatible with the clinical findings since the type of cell that this 'one process' is applied to will determine the rate of proliferation.

What is this 'one process'? It is the proliferation of CLL cells. Although it is right to think of CLL as a disease in which apoptosis fails, this alone would lead to a very benign condition with only the slow accumulation of malignant lymphocytes, similar to what is found in M-CLL. Progressive CLL requires excessive proliferation as well as deficient apoptosis. Orchard and Oscier (1996) found Ki-67 staining of peripheral blood lymphocytes to be up to tenfold higher in U-CLL than in M-CLL. Levels in bone marrow lymphocytes are higher, but the difference between M-CLL and U-CLL persists (Schrader et al. 2003). Ki-67 staining is at its highest in the proliferation centres (Moreton et al. 2003), which involve the interaction of CLL cells and CD4-positive T cells. The plentiful T cells in the proliferation centres are activated, expressing CD40 ligand and are attracted by the chemokines CCL17 and CCL22 that are secreted by CD40 ligand-stimulated CLL cells (Ghia et al. 2002). The chatter between T cells and B cells also upregulates survivin, one of the inhibitor of apoptosis proteins in the CLL cells (Granziero et al. 2001). Why this should be so in a tumour already expressing Mcl-1 and Bcl-2, is not clear; perhaps the cell is more vulnerable when dividing.

The proliferative history of the cell is reflected in the length of its telomeres. Damle et al. (2004) have demonstrated shorter telomeres and greater telomerase activity in cells from U-CLL than M-CLL, suggesting that the former is more proliferative than the latter. The greater number of cell divisions might account for the greater likelihood of accumulating deleterious chromosomal aberrations in this subset (Krober et al. 2002; Oscier et al. 2002).

We once described the CLL cells as partially activated, anergic and resistant to apoptosis (Caligaris-Cappio and Hamblin 1999). On the basis of what has gone before, we would expect M-CLL to be more anergic than U-CLL, the cell having emerged from a germinal centre before entering a proliferation centre. Experiments measuring the phosphorylation of tyrosine kinase following BCR stimulation tend to confirm this (Lanham et al. 2003). In U-CLL the CLL cell lacking this germinal centre-imposed order is decidedly friskier.

7
Surrogate Markers

IgV mutational analysis has enhanced our understanding of the biology of CLL, but it is also the most incisive prognostic tool that we have. Unfortunately, the technique is too complicated for most routine laboratories. A surrogate marker is required. Initially it seemed that expression of CD38 would provide the same information (Damle et al. 1999). A reproducible technique for its detection by flow cytometry has been described. Unfortunately, while it is a useful prognostic marker, it does not produce the same information as the mutational status of *IgV* genes (Hamblin et al. 2002; Krober et al. 2002). There is about 30% discordance between the two assays. Another disadvantage is that CD38 expression may change during the course of the disease (Hamblin et al. 2002). The usual reason for this is selection by chemotherapy, which tends to spare those cells expressing the most CD38.

It has been suggested that there are three patterns of CD38 expression: low, high and bimodal (Ghia et al. 2003). Only the last two are associated with disease progression, and only the last shows changes in expression as the proportion of cells with high expression of CD38 increases.

CD38 is a type II trans-membrane glycoprotein that acts as a complex ecto-enzyme with adenosine diphosphate (ADP)-ribosyl cyclase activity (Malavasi et al. 1994; Deaglio et al. 2001). In the B cell compartment CD38 is not a lineage marker, but it is expressed at times during B cell development when cell-to-cell interactions are crucial to development. Examples include an early bone marrow precursor cell, cells in the germinal centre and plasma cells. All the factors that signal its upregulation are as yet unknown, but they include both α- and γ-interferon (Bauvois et al. 1999). In patients with stage A CLL, raised CD38 expression is a better predictor of death from any cause than of death from CLL (Hamblin et al. 2002). Some patients with benign M-CLL with associated metastatic cancer had rising CD38 expression, the suggestion being that extraneous cytokines may affect the expression of CD38 on CLL cells, an event apparently demonstrated in a patient with CD38-positive CLL that became CD38 negative when chronic myelomonocytic leukaemia developed as a coexistent disease (Hamblin et al. 2002).

Why CD38 should be important in CLL is not clear, though it appears to have an indirect role in enhancing the signalling through the BCR (Deaglio et al. 2003; Lanham et al. 2003). The finding that *ZAP-70* was the gene that most clearly segregated the two subsets in the microarray experiments (Rosenwald et al. 2001) suggests a central role for signalling in the distinction of U-CLL and M-CLL.

The 70-kDa protein associated with the ζ-chain of the CD3 receptor of T cells (ZAP-70) is a member of the syk family of tyrosine kinases. ZAP-70 comprises three functional domains, two tandem src homology 2 (SH2) domains at the amino-terminus, a kinase domain at the carboxy-terminus, and a linker region called interdomain B, which connects the SH2 domain and the kinase domain. The two SH2 domains work co-operatively and bind with phosphorylated immunoreceptor tyrosine-based activation motifs (ITAM) of the T cell receptor ζ-chain, which further induces its own phosphorylation and activation (Kuroyama et al. 2004). For T cell signalling, collaboration between ZAP-70 and the other src kinases Lck and Fyn and members of the Tec kinase family leads to the activation of downstream signalling pathways including increases in calcium flux, protein kinase C, nuclear factor (NF) κB and Ras-mitogen activated protein (MAP) kinase activation and eventually to the activation of transcription factors that control the cell's response (Nel 2002).

As a rule, B cells lack ZAP-70 but use instead a related tyrosine kinase, syk, for signal transduction (Chan et al. 1994). ZAP-70 is, however, expressed through B cell early development and plays a role in the transition from pro-B to pre-B cells in the marrow (Schweighoffer et al. 2003). In experiments where the BCR of CLL cells was engaged with anti-IgM, there was phosphorylation of syk as an indicator of signal transduction. Most cases of M-CLL failed to signal, but those with U-CLL signalled normally (Chen et al. 2002; Lanham et al. 2003). Chen et al. (2002) detected ZAP-70 protein by immunoblotting in 12/12 cell lysates from cases of U-CLL, but in only 1/10 from cases of M-CLL. Phosphorylation of syk was greater in the ZAP-70-positive cases, and in these cases there was also phosphorylation of ZAP-70, which associated with the BCR within minutes of exposure to the anti-IgM. This suggests that ZAP-70 is involved in BCR signalling in U-CLL but not in M-CLL. A proportion of cases of M-CLL that do not signal via anti-IgM do signal when the BCR is engaged with either anti-IgD or anti-79a (Lanham et al. 2003; Stevenson and Caligaris-Cappio 2004). Zupo et al. (2000) had previously shown different responses of CD38-positive CLL cells when stimulated with anti-IgM and anti-IgD, the former leading to apoptosis, the latter protecting against it. Dissociation of anti-IgM and anti-CD79a or anti-CD79b responses is a feature of anergic B cells (Vilen et al. 2002).

Following their demonstration that *ZAP-70* was, as they put it "the best CLL subtype distinction gene" the NIH group used the Lymphochip technology to profile an expanded cohort of 107 patients (Wiestner et al. 2003). *ZAP-70* expression correctly predicted *IgV* mutation status in 93% of patients. Four patients with M-CLL had high *ZAP-70* expression and three with U-CLL had low *ZAP-70* expression. Both *ZAP-70* expression and *IgV* mutational status were equally able to predict time to requirement of treatment. They devised two simplified assays suitable for introduction into routine laboratories, though their quantitative reverse transcriptase polymerase chain reaction (RT-PCR) assay still required T cell depletion as a first step, and their immunohistochemical staining of bone marrow was only semi-quantitative.

A more suitable assay for routine laboratories has been devised independently by two groups. Crespo et al. (2003) used a flow cytometric technique to study a cohort of 56 patients with CLL, using an anti-CD3 counterstain to identify T cells. Taking a lower cut-off level of 20%, they found that all 21 patients with M-CLL had low levels of ZAP-70-positive cells and all but 3 of the 35 patients with U-CLL had high levels. As expected, ZAP-70 positivity predicted time to requirement of treatment and overall survival. Orchard et al. (2004) used a very similar assay, but relying on the greater intensity of staining to separate T cells and natural killer (NK) cells to study 167 patients with CLL. This time the lower cut-off was 10%. There were 13 (7.8%) discordant patients. Six of the 114 patients with M-CLL had high levels of ZAP-70; 7/53 with U-CLL had low levels of ZAP-70. Of the 6 discordant patients with M-CLL, 5 had between 97% and 98% sequence homology with the germline gene, and the other used the *V3-21* gene. Only one had a stable lymphocyte count. Of the 7 discordant patients with U-CLL, 2 had stable lymphocyte counts. Again the assay performed as well as *IgV* mutational status for predicting time to treatment and overall survival.

Flow cytometry for determination of ZAP-70 levels has obvious advantages over other assays, especially as it can be combined with diagnostic immunophenotyping. The assay works well on dimethylsulfoxide (DMSO) frozen cells and gives concordant results with gene expression assays. It is, however, not yet well established or quality-assured. Because the cells must be permeabilized prior to staining, some labs have had difficulties with the method. Only the Upstate antibody (clone 2F3.2) has been validated in published methods. Cross-reactivity with other tyrosine kinases may be a difficulty for other antibodies. Even in the most experienced hands, concordance with *IgV* mutations is not 100%. It is premature to abandon sequencing *IgV* genes for prognostic purposes.

A number of clinical trials are planned or under way making use of the new prognostic markers. The first question to be answered is whether 'watch and wait' is still a sensible strategy for early-stage CLL. The policy is based on a meta-analysis of clinical trials in which all stage A patients were randomized between early treatment with an alkylating agent and treatment delayed until progression occurred. We are now able to abstract a large proportion of patients who should never be treated, and we also have fludarabine-based treatments that are much more effective than chlorambucil. Clearly the question needs to be asked again.

Less obvious, but perhaps equally important, is the question as to whether some patients are treated unnecessarily. Although trials have suggested that Binet stage B and C patients benefit from treatment, and progressive stage A patients are nowadays also treated, I believe that some patients are still treated on the basis of a rising white cell count or the appearance of minor lymphadenopathy. Are some cases of M-CLL being treated inappropriately? Does such treatment hasten the appearance of immunodeficiency, autoimmunity or even Richter's syndrome? Trials are needed.

Acknowledgements I have received financial support for the many years that I have been studying CLL from Tenovus, the Leukaemia Research Fund and the Bournemouth Leukaemia Fund.

My thinking has been influenced on CLL by Prof. Freda Stevenson who has been a valued colleague, who has been my source of immunological knowledge and who had the foresight to set up the assay for immunoglobulin gene sequencing; by Dr. David Oscier, who has shared the clinical load with me for more than 20 years, who has been my guide in molecular matters, and who set up a chromosome laboratory to study CLL before almost anybody else; and by Dr. Jenny Orchard who has had day-to-day care of many of the patients and who has become a flow cytometry expert second to none. I am also indebted to the skill of Zadie Davis who has sequenced most of the genes, to Rachel Ibbotson who has operated the flow cytometer and to Anne Gardiner, Sarah Mould, and Sharron Glide who have done the karyotyping. Finally, I want to thank Prof. George Stevenson who was my mentor from the beginning and continues to give useful advice.

References

Albesiano E, Messmer BT, Damle RN, Allen SL, Rai KR, Chiorazzi N (2003) Activation-induced cytidine deaminase in chronic lymphocytic leukemia B cells: expression as multiple forms in a dynamic, variably sized fraction of the clone. Blood 102:3333–3339

Bahler DW, Aguilera NS, Chen CC, Abbondanzo SL, Swerdlow SH (2000) Histological and immunoglobulin VH gene analysis of interfollicular small lymphocytic lymphoma provides evidence for two types. Am J Pathol 157:1063–1070

Bauvois B, Durant L, Laboureau J, Barthelemy E, Rouillard D, Boulla G, Deterre P (1999) Upregulation of CD38 gene expression in leukemic B cells by interferon types I and II. J Interferon Cytokine Res 19:1059–1066

Bennett JM, Catovsky D, Daniel MT, Flandrin G, Galton DA, Gralnick HR, Sultan C (1989) French-American-British (FAB) Cooperative Group. Proposals for the classification of chronic (mature) B and T lymphoid leukaemias. J Clin Pathol 42:567–584

Berek C, Berger A, Apel M (1991) Maturation of the immune response in germinal centers. Cell 67:1121–1129

Brezinschek HP, Brezinschek RI, Dorner T, Lipsky PE (1998) Similar characteristics of the CDR3 of V(H)1-69/DP-10 rearrangements in normal human peripheral blood and chronic lymphocytic leukaemia blood cells. Br J Haematol 102:516–521

Broker BM, Klajman A, Youinou P, Jouquan J, Worman CP, Murphy J, Mackenzie L, Quarty-Papafio R, Blaschek M, Collins P (1988) Chronic lymphocytic leukemia (CLL) cells secrete multispecific autoantibodies. J Autoimmun 1:469–481

Caligaris-Cappio F (1996) Chronic lymphocytic leukemia: a malignancy of anti-self B-cells. Blood 67:2615–2620

Caligaris-Cappio F, Hamblin TJ (1999) B-cell chronic lymphocytic leukemia: a bird of a different feather. J Clin Oncol 17:399–408

Chan AC, van Oers NS, Tran A, Turka L, Law CL, Ryan JC, Clark EA, Weiss A (1994) Differential expression of ZAP-70 and Syk protein tyrosine kinases, and the role of this family of protein tyrosine kinases in TCR signaling. J Immunol 152:4758–4766

Chen L, Widhopf G, Huynh L, Rassenti L, Rai KR, Weiss A, Kipps TJ (2002) Expression of ZAP-70 is associated with increased B-cell receptor signaling in chronic lymphocytic leukemia. Blood 100:4069–4614

Chiorazzi N, Ferrarini M (2001) V gene mutations and CD38 expression define B-CLL subgroups. In: Cheson B (ed) Chronic lymphoid leukemias, 2nd edn. Marcel Dekker, New York, pp 81–109

Chiorazzi N, Ferrarini M (2003) B cell chronic lymphocytic leukemia: lessons learned from studies of the B cell receptor. Annu Rev Immunol 21:841–894

CLL Trialists' Collaborative Group (1999) Chemotherapeutic options in chronic lymphocytic leukemia: a meta-analysis of the randomised trials. J Natl Cancer Inst 91:861–868

Crespo M, Bosch F, Villamor N, Bellosillo B, Colomer D, Rozman M, Marce S, Lopez-Guillermo A, Campo E, Montserrat E (2003) ZAP-70 expression as a surrogate for immunoglobulin-variable-region mutations in chronic lymphocytic leukemia. N Engl J Med 348:1764–1775

Damle RN, Wasil T, Fais F, Ghiotto F, Valetto A, Allen SL, Buchbinder A, Budman D, Dittamr K, Kolitz J, Lichtman SM, Schulman P, Viciguerra VP, Rai KR, Ferrarini M, Chiorazzi N (1999) Ig V gene mutation status and CD38 expression as novel prognostic indicators in chronic lymphocytic leukemia. Blood 94:1840–1847

Damle RN, Batliwalla FM, Ghiotto F, Valetto A, Albesiano E, Sison C, Allen SL, Kolitz J, Vinciguerra VP, Kudalkar P, Wasil T, Rai KR, Ferrarini M, Gregersen PK, Chiorazzi N (2004) Telomere length and telomerase activity delineate distinctive replicative features of the B-CLL subgroups defined by immunoglobulin V gene mutations. Blood 103:375–382

Davis ZA, Orchard JA, Corcoran MM, Oscier DG (2003) Divergence from the germ-line sequence in unmutated chronic lymphocytic leukemia is due to somatic mutation rather than polymorphisms. Blood 102:3075

Deaglio S, Mehta K, Malavasi F (2001) Human CD38: a (r)evolutionary story of enzymes and receptors. Leuk Res 25:1–12

Deaglio S, Capobianco A, Bergui L, Durig J, Morabito F, Duhrsen U, Malavasi F (2003) CD38 is a signaling molecule in B-cell chronic lymphocytic leukemia cells. Blood 102:2146–2155

Deane M, Norton JD (1991) Preferential rearrangement of developmentally regulated immunoglobulin IgVH1 genes in human B-lineage leukaemias. Leukemia 5:646–650

Ebeling SB, Schutte MEM, Akkermans-Koolhaas KE, Bloem AC, Gmelig-Meyling FHJ, Logtenberg T (1992) Expression of members of the immunoglobulin VH-3 gene families is not restricted at the level of individual genes in human chronic lymphocytic leukemia. Int Immunol 4:313–320

Elison DG, Nathwani BN, Cho SY, Martin SE (1989) Interfollicular small lymphocytic lymphoma: the diagnostic significance of pseudofollicles. Hum Pathol 20:1108–1118

Fais F, Ghiotto F, Hashimoto S, Sellers B, Valetto A, Schulman P, Vinciguerra VP, Rai K, Rassenti LZ, Kipps TJ, Dighiero G, Schroeder HWJr, Ferrarini M, Chiorazzi N (1998) Chronic lymphocytic leukemia B cells express restricted sets of mutated and unmutated antigen receptors. J Clin Invest 102:1515–1525

Ghia P, Strola G, Granziero L, Geuna M, Guida G, Sallusto F, Ruffing N, Montagna L, Piccoli P, Chilosi M, Caligaris-Cappio F (2002) Chronic lymphocytic leukemia B cells are endowed with the capacity to attract CD4+, CD40L+ T cells by producing CCL22. Eur J Immunol 32:1403–1413

Ghia P, Guida G, Stella S, Gottardi D, Geuna M, Strola G, Scielzo C, Caligaris-Cappio F (2003) The pattern of CD38 expression defines a distinct subset of chronic lymphocytic leukemia (CLL) patients at risk of disease progression. Blood 101:1262–1269

Granziero L, Ghia P, Circosta P, Gottardi D, Strola G, Geuna M, Montagna L, Piccoli P, Chilosi M, Caligaris-Cappio F (2001) Survivin is expressed on CD40 stimulation and interfaces proliferation and apoptosis in B-cell chronic lymphocytic leukemia. Blood 97:2777–2783

Gurrieri C, McGuire P, Zan H, Yan XJ, Cerutti A, Albesiano E, Allen SL, Vinciguerra V, Rai KR, Ferrarini M, Casali P, Chiorazzi N (2002) Chronic lymphocytic leukemia B cells can undergo somatic hypermutation and intraclonal immunoglobin V(H)DJ(H) gene diversification, J Exp Med 196:629–639

Hamblin T (2002) Chronic lymphocytic leukaemia: one disease or two? Ann Hematol 81:299–303

Hamblin T, Davis Z, Gardiner A, Oscier DG, Stevenson FK (1999) Unmutated Ig V(H) genes are associated with a more aggressive form of chronic lymphocytic leukemia. Blood 94:1848–1854

Hamblin TJ, Orchard JA, Ibbotson RE, Davis Z, Thomas PW, Stevenson FK, Oscier DG (2002) CD38 expression and immunoglobulin variable region mutations are independent prognostic variables in chronic lymphocytic leukemia, but CD38 expression may vary during the course of the disease. Blood 99:1023–1029

Jacob J, Kelsoe G, Rajewsky K, Weiss U (1991) Intraclonal generation of antibody mutants in germinal centres. Nature 354:389–392

Jelinek DF, Tschumper RC, Geyer SM, Bone ND, Dewald GW, Hanson CA, Stenson MJ, Witzig TE, Tefferi A, Kay NE (2001) Analysis of clonal B-cell CD38 and immunoglobulin variable region sequence status in relation to clinical outcome for B-chronic lymphocytic leukaemia. Br J Haematol 115:854–861

Johnson TA, Rassenti LZ, Kipps TJ (1997) VH1 genes expressed in B cell chronic lymphocytic leukemia exhibits distinctive molecular features. J Immunol 158:235–246

Kipps TJ, Tomhave E, Pratt LF, Duffey S, Chen PP, Carson DA (1989) Developmentally restricted immunoglobulin heavy chain variable region gene expressed at high frequency in chronic lymphocytic leukemia. Proc Natl Acad Sci USA 86:5913–5917

Klein U, Tu Y, Stolovitzky GA, Mattioli M, Cattoretti G, Husson H, Freedman A, Inghirami G, Cro L, Baldini L, Neri A, Califano A, Dalla-Favera R (2001) Gene expression profiling of B cell chronic lymphocytic leukemia reveals a homogeneous phenotype related to memory B cells. J Exp Med 194:1625–1638

Krober A, Seiler T, Benner A, Bullinger L, Bruckle E, Lichter P, Dohner H, Stilgenbauer S (2002) V(H) mutation status, CD38 expression level, genomic aberrations, and survival in chronic lymphocytic leukemia. Blood 100:1410–1416

Kuroyama H, Ikeda T, Kasai M, Yamasaki S, Tatsumi M, Utsuyama M, Saito T, Hirokawa K (2004) Identification of a novel isoform of ZAP-70, truncated ZAP kinase. Biochem Biophys Res Commun 315:935–941

Lanham S, Hamblin TJ, Oscier DG, Stevenson FK, Packham G (2003) B-cell receptor signaling responsiveness correlates with VH gene mutational status on chronic lymphocytic leukemia. Blood 101:1087–1093

Lens SM, Keehnen RM, van Oers MH, van Lier RA, Pals ST, Koopman G (1996) Identification of a novel subpopulation of germinal center B cells characterized by expression of IgD and CD70. Eur J Immunol 26:1007–1011

Lin K, Sherrington PD, Dennis M, Matrai Z, Cawley JC, Pettitt AR (2002) Relationship between p53 dysfunction, CD38 expression, and IgV(H) mutation in chronic lymphocytic leukemia. Blood 100:1404–1409

MacLennan IC (1994) Germinal centers. Annu Rev Immunol 12:117–139

Malavasi F, Funaro A, Roggero S, Horenstein A, Calosso L, Mehta K (1994) Human CD38: a glycoprotein in search of a function. Immunol Today 15:95–97

Maloum K, Davi F, Merle-Beral H, Pritsch O, Magnac C, Vuillier F, Dighiero G, Troussard X, Mauro FF, Benichou J (2000) Expression of unmutated VH genes is a detrimental prognostic factor in chronic lymphocytic leukemia. Blood 95:377–378

Matrai Z, Sherrington PD, Pettitt AR, Zuzel M, Cawley JC (2003) CD38 expression in CLL is a marker of cell cycling. Blood 102:671a abstr 2482

Matutes E, Oscier D, Garcia-Marco-J, Ellis J, Copplestone A, Gillingham R, Hamblin T, Lens D, Swansbury GJ, Catovsky D (1996) Trisomy 12 defines a group of CLL with atypical morphology: correlation between cytogenetic, clinical and laboratory features in 544 patients. Br J Haematol 92:382–388

McCarthy H, Wierda WG, Barron LL, Cromwell CC, Wang J, Coombes KR, Rangel R, Elenitoba-Johnson KS, Keating MJ, Abruzzo LV (2003) High expression of activation-induced cytidine deaminase (AID) and splice variants is a distinctive feature of poor-prognosis chronic lymphocytic leukemia. Blood 101:4903–4908

Messmer BT, Ablesiano E, Massmer D, Chiorazzi N (2004) The pattern and distribution of immunoglobulin VH gene mutations in chronic lymphocytic leukemia B cells are consistent with the canonical somatic hypermutation process. Blood 103:3490–3495

Moreau EJ, Matutes E, A'Hern RP, Morilla AM, Morilla RM, Owusu-Ankomah KA, Seon BK, Catovsky D (1997) Improvement of the chronic lymphocytic leukemia scoring system with the monoclonal antibody SN8 (CD79b). Am J Clin Pathol 108:378–382

Moreton P, O'Connor S, Blythe D, Hillmen P, Jack AS (2003) The proliferating cells in CLL have a unique immunophenotype. Blood 102: suppl 1:187a abstr 652

Muramatsu M, Kinoshita K, Fagarasan S, Yamada S, Shinkai Y, Honjo T (2000) Class switch recombination and hypermutation require activation-induced cytidine deaminase (AID), a potential RNA editing enzyme. Cell 102:553–563

Nel AE (2002) T-cell activation through the antigen receptor. Part 1: signaling components, signaling pathways, and signal integration at he T-cell antigen receptor synapse. J Allergy Clin Immunol 109:758–770

Oppezzo P, Vuillier F, Vasconcelos Y, Dumas G, Magnac C, Payelle-Brogard B, Pritsch O, Dighiero G (2003) Chronic lymphocytic leukemia B cells expressing AID display dissociation between class switch recombination and somatic hypermutation. Blood 101:4029–4032

Orchard JA, Oscier DG (1996) Prognostic value of Ki 67 and cell cycle analysis in chronic lymphocytic leukaemia. Br J Haematol 93:116

Orchard JA, Ibbotson RE, Davis Z, Wiestner A, Rosenwald A, Thomas PW, Hamblin TJ, Staudt LM, Oscier DG (2004) ZAP-70 expression and prognosis in chronic lymphocytic leukaemia. Lancet 363:105–111

Oscier DG, Thompsett A, Zhu D, Stevenson FK (1997) Differential rates of somatic hypermutation in VH genes among subsets of chronic lymphocytic leukemia defined by chromosomal abnormalities. Blood 89:4153–4160

Oscier DG, Gardiner AC, Mould SJ, Glide S, Davies Z, Ibbotson RE, Corcoran MM, Chapman RM, Thomas PW, Copplestone JA, Orchard JA, Hamblin TJ (2002) Multivariate analysis of prognostic factors in CLL: clinical stage, IGVH gene mutational status, and loss or mutation of the p53 gene are independent prognostic factors. Blood 100:1177–1184

Potter KN, Orchard J, Critchley E, Mockridge CI, Jose A, Stevenson FK (2003) Features of the overexpressed V1-69 genes in the unmutated subset of chronic lymphocytic leukemia are distinct from those in the healthy elderly repertoire. Blood 101:3082–3084

Ritgen M, Lange A, Stilgenbauer S, Dohner H, Bretscher C, Bosse H, Stuhr A, Kneba M, Dreger P (2003) Unmutated immunoglobulin variable heavy-chain gene status remains an adverse prognostic factor after autologous stem cell transplantation for chronic lymphocytic leukemia. Blood 101:2049–2053

Rosenwald A, Alizadeh AA, Widhopf G, Simon R, Davis RE, Yu X, Yang L, Pickeral OK, Rassenti LZ, Powell J, Botstein D, Byrd JC, Grever MR, Cheson BD, Chiorazzi N, Wilson WH, Kipps TJ, Brown PO, Staudt LM (2001) Relation of gene expression phenotype to immunoglobulin mutation genotype in B cell chronic lymphocytic leukemia. J Exp Med 194:1639–1647

Rawstron AC, Green MJ, Kuzmicki A, Kennedy B, Fenton JA, Evans PA, O'Connor SJ, Richards SJ, Morgan GJ, Jack AS, Hillmen P (2002) Monoclonal B lymphocytes with the characteristics of "indolent" chronic lymphocytic leukemia are present in 3.5% of adults with normal blood counts. Blood 100:635–639

Schmid C, Isaacson PG (1994) Proliferation centres in B-cell malignant lymphoma, lymphocytic (B-CLL): an immunophenotypic study. Histopathology 24:445–451

Schrader C, Tiemann M, Karimi S, Janssen D, Stilgenbauer S, Doener H, Parwaresch R, Dreger P, Kneba M, Ritgen M (2003) Ki-67 expression in chronic lymphocytic leukemia: a prognostic marker and indicator for unmutated immunoglobulin heavy-chain variable region. Blood 102:666a abstr 2467

Schroeder HW Jr, Dighiero G (1994) The pathogenesis of chronic lymphocytic leukemia: analysis of the antibody repertoire. Immunol Today 15:288–294

Schweighoffer E, Vanes L, Mathiot A, Nakamura T, Tybulewicz VL (2003) Unexpected requirement for ZAP-70 in pre-B cell development and allelic exclusion. Immunity 18:523–533

Silverman GJ (1997) B-cell superantigens. Immunol Today 18:379–386

Stevenson FK, Caligaris-Cappio (2004) Chronic lymphocytic leukemia: revelations from the B-cell receptor. Blood 103:4389–4395

Tobin G, Thunberg U, Johnson A, Thorn I, Soderberg O, Hultdin M, Botling J, Enblad G, Sallstrom J, Sundstrom C, Roos G, Rosenquist R (2002) Somatically mutated IgVH3-21 genes characterize a new subset of chronic lymphocytic leukemia. Blood 99:2262–2264

Tobin G, Thunberg U, Johnson A, Eriksson I, Soderberg O, Karlsson K, Merup M, Juliusson G, Vilpo J, Enblad G, Sundstrom C, Roos G, Rosenquist R (2003) Chronic lymphocytic leukemias utilizing the VH3-21 gene display highly restricted Vlambda2-14 gene use and homologous CDR3s: implicating recognition of a common antigen epitope. Blood 101:4952–4957

Toellner KM, Jenkinson WE, Taylor DR, Khan M, Sze DM, Sansom DM, Vinuesa CG, MacLennan IC (2002) Low-level hypermutation in T cell-independent germinal centers compared with high mutation rates associated with T cell-dependent germinal centers. J Exp Med 195:383–389

van Oers MH, Pals ST, Evers LM, van der Schoot CE, Koopman G, Bonfrer JM, Hintzen RQ, von dem Borne AE, van Lier RA (1993) Expression and release of CD27 in human B-cell malignancies. Blood 82:3430–3436

Vilen BJ, Burke KM, Sleater M, Cambier JC (2002) Transmodulation of BCR signaling by transduction-incompetent antigen receptors: implications for impaired signaling in anergic B cells. J Immunol 168:4344–4351

Weller S, Faili A, Garcia C, Braun MC, Le Deist FF, de Saint Basile GG, Hermine O, Fischer A, Reynaud CA, Weill JC (2001) CD40-CD40L independent Ig gene hypermutation suggests a second B cell diversification pathway in humans. Proc Natl Acad Sci U S A 98:1166–1170

Wiestner A, Rosenwald A, Barry TS, Wright G, Davis RE, Henrickson SE, Zhao H, Ibbotson RE, Orchard JA, Davis Z, Stetler-Stevenson M, Raffeld M, Arthur DC, Marti GE, Wilson WH, Hamblin TJ, Oscier DG, Staudt LM (2003) ZAP-70 expression identifies a chronic lymphocytic leukemia subtype with unmutated immunoglobulin genes, inferior clinical outcome, and distinct gene expression profile. Blood 101:4944–4951

Zhu D, Hawkins RE, Hamblin TJ, Stevenson FK (1974) Clonal history of a human follicular lymphoma as revealed in the immunoglobulin variable region genes. Br J Haematol 86:505–512

Zhu D, McCarthy H, Ottensmeier CH, Johnson P, Hamblin TJ, Stevenson FK (2002) Acquisition of potential N-glycosylation sites in the immunoglobulin variable region by somatic mutation is a distinctive feature of follicular lymphoma. Blood 99:2562–2568

Zupo S, Massara R, Dono M, Rossi E, Malavasi F, Cosulich ME, Ferrarini M (2002) Apoptosis or plasma cell differentiation of CD38-positive-B-chronic lymphocytic leukemia cells induced by cross-linking of surface IgM or IgD. Blood 95:1199–1206

Subject Index

Current Topics in Microbiology and Immunology

Volumes published since 1989 (and still available)

Vol. 249: **Jones, Peter A.; Vogt, Peter K. (Eds.):** DNA Methylation and Cancer. 2000. 16 figs. IX, 169 pp. ISBN 3-540-66608-7

Vol. 250: **Aktories, Klaus; Wilkins, Tracy, D. (Eds.):** Clostridium difficile. 2000. 20 figs. IX, 143 pp. ISBN 3-540-67291-5

Vol. 251: **Melchers, Fritz (Ed.):** Lymphoid Organogenesis. 2000. 62 figs. XII, 215 pp. ISBN 3-540-67569-8

Vol. 252: **Potter, Michael; Melchers, Fritz (Eds.):** B1 Lymphocytes in B Cell Neoplasia. 2000. XIII, 326 pp. ISBN 3-540-67567-1

Vol. 253: **Gosztonyi, Georg (Ed.):** The Mechanisms of Neuronal Damage in Virus Infections of the Nervous System. 2001. approx. XVI, 270 pp. ISBN 3-540-67617-1

Vol. 254: **Privalsky, Martin L. (Ed.):** Transcriptional Corepressors. 2001. 25 figs. XIV, 190 pp. ISBN 3-540-67569-8

Vol. 255: **Hirai, Kanji (Ed.):** Marek's Disease. 2001. 22 figs. XII, 294 pp. ISBN 3-540-67798-4

Vol. 256: **Schmaljohn, Connie S.; Nichol, Stuart T. (Eds.):** Hantaviruses. 2001. 24 figs. XI, 196 pp. ISBN 3-540-41045-7

Vol. 257: **van der Goot, Gisou (Ed.):** PoreForming Toxins, 2001. 19 figs. IX, 166 pp. ISBN 3-540-41386-3

Vol. 258: **Takada, Kenzo (Ed.):** Epstein-Barr Virus and Human Cancer. 2001. 38 figs. IX, 233 pp. ISBN 3-540-41506-8

Vol. 259: **Hauber, Joachim, Vogt, Peter K. (Eds.):** Nuclear Export of Viral RNAs. 2001. 19 figs. IX, 131 pp. ISBN 3-540-41278-6

Vol. 260: **Burton, Didier R. (Ed.):** Antibodies in Viral Infection. 2001. 51 figs. IX, 309 pp. ISBN 3-540-41611-0

Vol. 261: **Trono, Didier (Ed.):** Lentiviral Vectors. 2002. 32 figs. X, 258 pp. ISBN 3-540-42190-4

Vol. 262: **Oldstone, Michael B.A. (Ed.):** Arenaviruses I. 2002. 30 figs. XVIII, 197 pp. ISBN 3-540-42244-7

Vol. 263: **Oldstone, Michael B. A. (Ed.):** Arenaviruses II. 2002. 49 figs. XVIII, 268 pp. ISBN 3-540-42705-8

Vol. 264/I: **Hacker, Jörg; Kaper, James B. (Eds.):** Pathogenicity Islands and the Evolution of Microbes. 2002. 34 figs. XVIII, 232 pp. ISBN 3-540-42681-7

Vol. 264/II: **Hacker, Jörg; Kaper, James B. (Eds.):** Pathogenicity Islands and the Evolution of Microbes. 2002. 24 figs. XVIII, 228 pp. ISBN 3-540-42682-5

Vol. 265: **Dietzschold, Bernhard; Richt, Jürgen A. (Eds.):** Protective and Pathological Immune Responses in the CNS. 2002. 21 figs. X, 278 pp. ISBN 3-540-42668X

Vol. 266: **Cooper, Koproski (Eds.):** The Interface Between Innate and Acquired Immunity, 2002. 15 figs. XIV, 116 pp. ISBN 3-540-42894-X

Vol. 267: **Mackenzie, John S.; Barrett, Alan D. T.; Deubel, Vincent (Eds.):** Japanese Encephalitis and West Nile Viruses. 2002. 66 figs. X, 418 pp. ISBN 3-540-42783X

Vol. 268: **Zwickl, Peter; Baumeister, Wolfgang (Eds.):** The Proteasome-Ubiquitin Protein Degradation Pathway. 2002. 17 figs. X, 213 pp. ISBN 3-540-43096-2

Vol. 269: **Koszinowski, Ulrich H.; Hengel, Hartmut (Eds.):** Viral Proteins Counteracting Host Defenses. 2002. 47 figs. XII, 325 pp. ISBN 3-540-43261-2

Vol. 270: **Beutler, Bruce; Wagner, Hermann (Eds.):** Toll-Like Receptor Family

Members and Their Ligands. 2002. 31 figs. X, 192 pp. ISBN 3-540-43560-3

Vol. 271: **Koehler, Theresa M. (Ed.):** Anthrax. 2002. 14 figs. X, 169 pp. ISBN 3-540-43497-6

Vol. 272: **Doerfler, Walter; Böhm, Petra (Eds.):** Adenoviruses: Model and Vectors in Virus-Host Interactions. Virion and Structure, Viral Replication, Host Cell Interactions. 2003. 63 figs., approx. 280 pp. ISBN 3-540-00154-9

Vol. 273: **Doerfler, Walter; Böhm, Petra (Eds.):** Adenoviruses: Model and Vectors in VirusHost Interactions. Immune System, Oncogenesis, Gene Therapy. 2004. 35 figs., approx. 280 pp. ISBN 3-540-06851-1

Vol. 274: **Workman, Jerry L. (Ed.):** Protein Complexes that Modify Chromatin. 2003. 38 figs., XII, 296 pp. ISBN 3-540-44208-1

Vol. 275: **Fan, Hung (Ed.):** Jaagsiekte Sheep Retrovirus and Lung Cancer. 2003. 63 figs., XII, 252 pp. ISBN 3-540-44096-3

Vol. 276: **Steinkasserer, Alexander (Ed.):** Dendritic Cells and Virus Infection. 2003. 24 figs., X, 296 pp. ISBN 3-540-44290-1

Vol. 277: **Rethwilm, Axel (Ed.):** Foamy Viruses. 2003. 40 figs., X, 214 pp. ISBN 3-540-44388-6

Vol. 278: **Salomon, Daniel R.; Wilson, Carolyn (Eds.):** Xenotransplantation. 2003. 22 figs., IX, 254 pp. ISBN 3-540-00210-3

Vol. 279: **Thomas, George; Sabatini, David; Hall, Michael N. (Eds.):** TOR. 2004. 49 figs., X, 364 pp. ISBN 3-540-00534X

Vol. 280: **Heber-Katz, Ellen (Ed.):** Regeneration: Stem Cells and Beyond. 2004. 42 figs., XII, 194 pp. ISBN 3-540-02238-4

Vol. 281: **Young, John A. T. (Ed.):** Cellular Factors Involved in Early Steps of Retroviral Replication. 2003. 21 figs., IX, 240 pp. ISBN 3-540-00844-6

Vol. 282: **Stenmark, Harald (Ed.):** Phosphoinositides in Subcellular Targeting and Enzyme Activation. 2003. 20 figs., X, 210 pp. ISBN 3-540-00950-7

Vol. 283: **Kawaoka, Yoshihiro (Ed.):** Biology of Negative Strand RNA Viruses: The Power of Reverse Genetics. 2004. 24 figs., IX, 350 pp. ISBN 3-540-40661-1

Vol. 284: **Harris, David (Ed.):** Mad Cow Disease and Related Spongiform Encephalopathies. 2004. 34 figs., IX, 219 pp. ISBN 3-540-20107-6

Vol. 285: **Marsh, Mark (Ed.):** Membrane Trafficking in Viral Replication. 2004. 19 figs., IX, 259 pp. ISBN 3-540-21430-5

Vol. 286: **Madshus, Inger H. (Ed.):** Signalling from Internalized Growth Factor Receptors. 2004. 19 figs., IX, 187 pp. ISBN 3-540-21038-5

Vol. 287: **Enjuanes, Luis (Ed.):** Coronavirus Replication and Reverse Genetics. 2005. 49 figs., XI, 257 pp. ISBN 3-540-21494-1

Vol. 288: **Mahy, Brain W. J. (Ed.):** Foot-and-Mouth-Disease Virus. 2005. 16 figs., IX, 178 pp. ISBN 3-540-22419X

Vol. 289: **Griffin, Diane E. (Ed.):** Role of Apoptosis in Infection. 2005. 40 figs., IX, 294 pp. ISBN 3-540-23006-8

Vol. 290: **Singh, Harinder; Grosschedl, Rudolf (Eds.):** Molecular Analysis of B Lymphocyte Development and Activation. 2005. 28 figs., XI, 255 pp. ISBN 3-540-23090-4

Vol. 291: **Boquet, Patrice; Lemichez Emmanuel (Eds.)** Bacterial Virulence Factors and Rho GTPases. 2005. 28 figs., IX, 196 pp. ISBN 3-540-23865-4

Vol. 292: **Fu, Zhen F (Ed.):** The World of Rhabdoviruses. 2005. 27 figs., X, 210 pp. ISBN 3-540-24011-X

Vol. 293: **Kyewski, Bruno; Suri-Payer, Elisabeth (Eds.):** CD4+CD25+ Regulatory T Cells: Origin, Function and Therapeutic Potential. 2005. 22 figs., XII, 332 pp. ISBN 3-540-24444-1

Printing: Krips bv, Meppel
Binding: Stürtz, Würzburg